SPIRAL UP YOGA

SPIRAL UP YOGA

Five Minutes Per Day Lifelong Self-Care
Foundation for Body, Mind and Soul

John E. Groberg

The flexible are preserved unbroken.
The bent become straight.
The empty are filled.
The exhausted become renewed.
The poor are enriched.
The rich are confounded.
- LAO TZU

DEDICATION

This book is dedicated to our collective disillusionment; to the piercing of all illusions which we continue to operate under and lend our belief to, that keep us from seeing divine perfection everywhere and in everyone, including ourselves.

ACKNOWLEDGEMENTS

I would like to acknowledge the contributions of several individuals who have helped make this book possible.

To Beverly Groberg, for not giving up on me or insisting that I get a real job, even though I'm sure that would have been more comforting at times. Thank you for your patience, support and faith in me. Thank you for being a fantastic mother to our amazing six children. You're already making a bigger difference in the world than you could know. Thank you also for being my gorgeous model and the face of Spiral Up Yoga. I love you as completely as I currently know how, and I look forward to experiencing how our love continues to evolve in the years, decades and eons ahead.

To my parents, John H. Groberg and Jean Groberg, thank you for all your sacrifices, efforts and service, known and unknown to me, and for your ongoing example of what an inspired life of service to family, church and community looks like.

To Master Alex Lee, my first yoga instructor and personal coach. Thank you for being a model of what enlightened living looks and feels like in body, in mind, and in soul. Thank you for helping me to see the importance of involving the body in any form of lasting spiritual growth.

To Steve Chandler, master coach and colleague. Thank you for helping me to see the more immediate possibilities of what I had in Spiral Up Yoga and inspiring me to not wait on anyone else's permission, and to "ship it." Thank you also for many years of insight and clarity through your books and coaching.

To Michael Neill, Supercoach and mentor. Thank you for training me in the ways of a Supercoach and for your example of what is possible when it comes to helping people transform their lives by seeing more clearly the nature of our humanity.

To countless authors over the past millennia, and also contemporary to me, who have written truly lasting works that have inspired and instructed me in the nature of Life. As an author myself now, I have a newfound appreciation of you beyond what I had as a reader, and my respect for you has deepened even more.

Finally, to you, the reader of this book. I acknowledge you as a divine being having a human experience. I appreciate your willingness to buy this book and read it and test it out for yourself. I promise you that as you do test it out in your own life, your personal experience of life will be transformed in small and great ways that are too many to enumerate. May the superior version of yourself that evolves from your consistent practice of Spiral Up Yoga be an inspiration to others in your life and a greater source of joy in yours.

TABLE OF CONTENTS

MEDICAL DISCLAIMER

This book does contain instructions for doing physical body work. As with all physical body work that you undertake, you should do so with carefulness and mindfulness. If you have any medical conditions or injuries, please use your own best judgment and consult a medical doctor before engaging in the physical body work. The author is not responsible for any choices you make and I obviously cannot know what your current physical condition is. I am not a medical doctor (or any other type of doctor) and am not giving you medical advice.

FOREWORD: HOW TO SET YOURSELF FREE

"The spiral is a spiritualized circle.
In the spiral form, the circle, uncoiled,
has ceased to be vicious; it has been set free."
~ Vladimir Nabokov, Speak, Memory

There aren't many ideas in modern day life that are truly and accurately described as revolutionary—but here, in this book, is one.

What if your yoga practice could always be a daily practice, even if you only had five minutes to give to it? What if the burdensome time and calendar element were eliminated altogether?

When I first heard John Groberg describe his discovery and invention to me, I was immediately skeptical. It sounded gimmicky and too good to be true.

I did know the problem he was trying to solve was a real problem. Most people I knew who did yoga had very full lives and had a hard time fitting their yoga practice and classes into their calendars. Then, after they missed a week or two, they would become disheartened and the practice would fade.

John Groberg's system solved that problem. You could do it in your home. You could even do it in five minutes if that's all you had. You could stay continuously connected and committed to your practice without any challenges from your calendar. Really?

And then came the part that convinced me. John had been using this practice himself for a long, long time. It was an experiment he performed on himself to solve his own problem with keeping his practice consistent.

Then John proved the power of his discovery further to me when he put on a special demonstration of it for me and a large group of my clients who were meeting in Chicago. We all got up early in the morning and met in the conference room before the meeting was to begin. We wore loose clothing and were ready for anything.

John stood in front of us and gave a mesmerizing, persuasive talk about what yoga was, the spiritual, mental and physical benefits of it, and how he had developed his system. You'll read all about that in this interesting book. He touches all the bases. His lifetime of deep study into personal growth and spirituality is reflected here.

He then took us through a series of short but very satisfying exercises. We were twisting, stretching, and breathing deeply as he explained the process. Even those of us who had never done yoga felt refreshed and peacefully excited at the conclusion of our time.

Nabokov's quote at the beginning of this piece refers to a vicious circle we all know about. It's the trapped, groundhog day spinning we do when our power stops evolving and we are living robotically. Same old same old. It's that circular rut we get into. And, as they say, the only difference between a rut and a grave is a few feet.

Groberg's system of practice gives us the freedom to spiral up. It gives us a way to connect daily to that higher Self inside us that refreshes all creativity and spirit. It's one thing to ponder spiritual concepts with the mind, but it's quite another to unify mind, body and spirit in movement and exercise. It's the difference between thinking and being.

There is even better news than what I have written about so far. Of course, it is a truly revolutionary thing to have invented a way for yoga practitioners to ensure that they can now do it daily, in short periods of time if need be.

But this book goes far deeper than that. It is a rich compendium of John Groberg's entire life study on how to be effective and fulfilled as a spiritual being making a difference in the world. Not only is this book about how to do yoga, but it is also about how to have your yoga practice stand as a microcosm for the bigger picture… the good life itself.

Here we are introduced to living in flow… not in abrupt starts and stops. As John explains, the more we cultivate this flow mode, the more we are experiencing happiness in the present moment, and a positive vision for the future. And because he gives is an amazingly thorough Whole Life lesson in these pages, this book will reach people way beyond the subject of yoga. This short, compact book is bound to also become a classic in the category of personal growth and self-help.

This, to me, is as good a field manual for a fulfilling life as I have read in many a year. It is user-friendly and immediately applicable to anyone and everyone's life. It truly liberates you from the vicious circle that keeps so many people feeling stuck.

Sharing his personal discovery and method for daily rejuvenation will go down as one of the finest acts of generosity ever expressed in the world of books and media, so you might want to share this book with friends and family (and all people caught in the circle). Now it's time to enjoy it for yourself (as you certainly will).

Steve Chandler
Phoenix, Arizona, February, 2012

INTRODUCTION

. . . .

THE UNPLANNED YOGA BOOK

The book you now hold in your hands is not just a yoga book. There are plenty of those already written by people much more expert in yoga than I. This book is actually a personal invitation to undertake, in a new and more comprehensive way, the greatest treasure hunt there is in life – the rediscovery and realization of your true self (or soul) and the bringing forth of it more abundantly into your daily living and being. It is also a map I've drawn to help you navigate the territory with more clarity and ease, and a simple daily system that takes five minutes or less per day to stay on course in this amazing journey.

I didn't plan on writing a yoga book. I planned to write about such things as transforming your life, seeing with greater clarity, deepening your relationships, raising children with more joy and ease, and generally increasing your well-being and peace of mind regardless of your circumstances. Yet here it is, my first published work, called Spiral Up Yoga. How did this happen? Let me explain. I think it will be useful to you as you undertake reading and testing this book in your own life.

All my life I have been an avid student of the human experience. I have read hundreds of books from some of the greatest authors throughout time. I have always been attracted to the timeless – to books that transcend time and place and illuminate the path of the human condition. Books that are just as relevant to the reader today as they were thousands of years ago and as they will be thousands of years from now.

As time passed I felt an undeniable desire, almost a duty, to go beyond consuming such books and to create my own; to contribute a little something to the great library of life as a way of showing my gratitude for all those who contributed so powerfully before me. But while I had lots of ideas and a long list of possible book subjects and titles, something was missing still.

UNDERSTANDING VS. REALIZING

One of my early realizations was that understanding things was really just kindergarten. There is a big difference between understanding something and realizing it. To understand is to have an intellectual grasp of a principle that you can explain in words. To realize is to make it real in your life; not just a theory or a belief, but your reality – your actual way of seeing and being. So many of the great books that I had read and cherished were, at the end of the day, mostly intellectual understandings to me. I had no doubt that they sprang from actual realizations of the author, but those realizations could not really be transmitted in the written word. For them to become my own realizations, I would have to make the same journey within myself that the authors had, and discover for myself the same truths they did.

THE TAO

The great Lao Tzu wrote over 2,500 years ago in the Tao te Ching, 67th verse, these lines that I love:

> *"All the world talks about my Tao with such familiarity — what folly! The Tao is not something found at the marketplace, or passed from father to son. It is not something gained by knowing or lost by forgetting. If the Tao were like this, it would have been lost and forgotten long ago."*

The Tao (pronounced "dow") means the way of virtue, or as I have come to see it, the way of the soul or the innate nature of the soul. It can be written about, but it cannot be purchased in the marketplace. A father can teach it to his son, but only the son can make the journey within himself to make it real for him. Studying it cannot make it yours, because knowledge is not enough. Forgetting it doesn't mean it is lost, because it resides eternally within each one of us as the great treasure of life, as the kingdom of heaven within, just waiting to be re-discovered by each individual personality.

YOGA AND THE TAO

> **The Tao is the way of the soul. Yoga is the way to the soul.**

Until I discovered yoga for myself and started practicing it, I didn't realize how it fit into the Tao. Some seven years later, I now realize that:

The Tao is the way <u>of</u> the soul. Yoga is the way <u>to</u> the soul.

That's a pretty bold statement, but one I am very comfortable making. Yoga, when properly understood, is much more than a form of exercise involving stretching and balancing in strange positions. Yoga literally means "union" of body, mind and soul. I take that definition quite broadly. To me, anything that helps me to unify my body, mind, and soul is yoga. The physical postures that most people think of when they think of yoga are just one form of yoga (albeit an important one). But without the proper intention of unifying body, mind, and soul, the yoga postures are not really yoga – they are just stretching exercises.

I first discovered yoga in 2005. My first yoga instructor was an incredible man named Alex Lee. He was from Korea and his English was rudimentary, but I could tell right away that he was a living model of someone who had realized the Tao in his own life and was living it. He was both kind and incisive, both flexible and strong, both yin and yang. I remember him telling me on several occasions something like this (these are not his exact words, just my recollection):

> *"You know too much. Knowing not enough. All your knowing leaves you with this! [He slaps my inflexible and out of balance body]. The soul cannot be realized through mind only. Many think they know truth and preach they know truth, but their bodies tell otherwise. Their bodies tell truth. A person who studies whole life all the great spiritual texts, but body is stiff and head is hot, this person knows much but realizes little. A person who has through the body obtained self-realization, though they never once read any scripture, will already know the true meaning of all scripture."*

At first, I thought this was harsh and not right, but he didn't care if I agreed with him. With time, I began to see some of what he meant. I began to see how I couldn't really compartmentalize my spiritual life to the mind and reserve exercise for the physical body. This is primarily how the western world sees things; exercise is for the body and spirituality is for the mind and heart, and the two are quite separate endeavors. It is true that one can exercise and maintain the body well and not be spiritual at all. It is also true that one can pursue a spiritual life through the study of scriptures and understand many things, but still allow the body to become stiff, inflamed, and out of balance. But is exercise only for the body that neglects the soul, true health? Is spiritual study for the mind and soul that neglects the body, true spirituality? I began to see that both ways were incomplete and that even pursuing both ways at the same time, but compartmentalized and separate, was still incomplete. There was a synergy to unifying the simultaneous development of body, mind, and soul that in the western mindset, which I was raised with, was missing – a synergy that I now see is the key to true well-being of body, mind and soul.

I have since come to see that master Lee was really saying the same thing as Lao Tzu in the passage I quoted earlier; that true realization of who we really are is not something that can be gained by knowing, nor is it something that can be lost by forgetting. The kingdom of heaven truly is within us already, as Jesus taught. But it is covered up by multiple layers of illusions of the mind and walls of tension in the body. To discover the kingdom of heaven within, which is to say to discover and allow the true nature of our souls to shine forth, we must each individually learn to uncover our divinity by seeing through the illusions in our mind and dissolving the tension in our bodies. This uncovering work cannot be done through scholarly study alone; and in fact scholarly study often becomes a detour and an avoidance of the real work, which is done in the body and in the realm of behavior.

THE SEVEN WINDOWS TO THE SOUL

As I began to practice yoga and meditation and learn about the energy body and chakra system, it became clear to me that our energy body and its seven major chakras are the keys to unlocking a fuller expression of our souls, living in the Tao, and realizing the kingdom of heaven within. Each chakra is like one of seven windows to the soul. We are all born with those windows clear and with the light of the soul shining through them. But over time, the windows begin to collect dust in the form of illusions that we believe or adopt from others. The longer that dust goes without being cleaned away, the thicker it gets and it even begins to calcify and become crusty. As it does, the light of the soul becomes more and more obscured from our awareness. It's always there, shining as bright as ever, but we just don't notice it through the thickly crusted-over windows. The crustiness first shows up as the experience of stress, guilt, shame, worry, and insecurity in our minds, and ultimately develops into tension, stiffness, imbalance, and disease in our physical bodies. Therefore, it is pretty clear to me that any effort to clean off these windows must certainly include, and may even begin with, body work.

As I continued to practice yoga, I began to recover lost flexibility and fluidity throughout my body, but the benefits were far beyond physical. I noticed that without really trying, I had a greater sense of mental well-being, less judgment of myself and others, more patience, and it was generally becoming harder and harder to get upset over things that happened differently than I expected.

DIVINE. ALIGN. SHINE.

One day, while I was taking a shower, the following three words came into my mind very clearly – almost as if spoken or seen:

Divine. Align. Shine.

It's hard to describe, but it was very clear to me that these three words were a simple formula for all personal growth. It all begins by realizing for ourselves – not just intellectually, but through direct personal experience – that we are, at our essence, divine beings. Realizing this truth, though, is not enough. We must continually align and realign ourselves to this divinity, and as we do, the light of our divinity will naturally shine forth from us, expressing its innumerable innate qualities including love, service, valor, patience, fearlessness, resiliency, trust, peace, and joy. The human condition is such that this alignment with our divinity is easily lost, almost on a daily basis, like dust collecting on a window. If we don't develop a daily practice of self-care that cleans away this dust and realigns us with our divinity, it's not long before the light dims and life looks bleak. This daily realigning process is really what Spiral Up Yoga is all about.

MAKING YOGA ACCESSIBLE AND PRACTICAL FOR ALL

After practicing yoga for some time, I realized for myself that yoga can create this realigning and unifying of body, mind and soul. Many thousands of years of history confirmed to me that this was a timeless, tangible practice that really made a difference in one's experience of life. The challenge, I discovered, is that as it is typically practiced, yoga is just not practical to be a daily practice for most people, certainly not for me. Beyond that, it is seen by many as mostly a feminine form of exercise and stretching, or only for young, in-shape people, and is therefore never explored by many. My personal journey in creating Spiral Up Yoga was to solve these challenges, and now that I have, my desire is to share it with as many others as I can reach, and this book is the beginning of doing that.

LIFE COACHING

Beyond teaching a specific five-minute-a-day system for bringing the power of yoga into your daily life, this book also contains many of the principles and realizations that I have personally gained through my practice of yoga and also through my experience as a trans-formational life coach working with clients to help them see their lives with greater clarity. In this book, I share many things that I'm certain you won't find in any other book about yoga. In many ways this book is more about life coaching than it is about doing yoga poses. I've found that life coaching, at its best, is really about re-discovering lost and forgotten aspects of your soul, and using the power of working in a coaching relationship to help bring more of those aspects or qualities into your daily life.

The seven chakras of the energy body turn out to be the perfect organizing system for going about the inner work of re-discovering and releasing your soul's full potential. Each of the seven chakras deals with different qualities of the soul that are either allowed to be expressed as that chakra is opened and strengthened, or suppressed as that chakra is covered up in dust and crustiness. So as I went about writing about the seven chakras and their individual meaning and characteristics, the life coaching principles that applied most to the qualities of each chakra just naturally fell together. Even if you never do the physical body work portion of the Spiral Up Yoga system, you will still be able to benefit tremendously from the life coaching principles, distinctions, and analogies I share. But if you want to take this beyond intellectual understanding, to your own personal realizing embodiment, you'll need to do the physical body work too, and not make this like reading most other books – just another mental consumption that may educate your mind but doesn't really transform your life. The good news is the whole point of the Spiral Up Yoga system is to make the physical body work extremely simple, easy, and immediately reward-ing to do just a few minutes every day.

THIS BOOK WILL NOT TRANSFORM YOU

This book will not transform you. It will not change your life. It doesn't have that kind of power. Neither does any other book. The only power this or any book has is to point you in the direction of the source of your transformation, and that source is within you – your very own soul. This book is written as a personal invitation to uncover and re-discover aspects of your soul that are currently obscured by years of sedimentary crustiness. The simple five-minute-a-day system organized around the seven chakras tied to the seven days of the week is presented as an unforgettably simple structure that I invite you to adopt, and from it create your own personalized daily self-care practice. Sticking with this simple daily practice and evolving it as you evolve is what will allow you to scrape away the sediment and clean off the seven windows of your soul, and that is what will transform you and change your life forever.

POSTCARDS FROM BEYOND THE VEIL OF ILLUSION

I have included in this book some of my favorite quotes from some of my favorite authors. The authors I have selected are ones who have personally made their own journey within and have pierced the veil of illusion behind which most of us still live. The messages they communicate in these quotes are like postcards sent to us from the other side of the veil of illusion. They are really just describing what things look like without illusions distorting them. Even though they may seem lofty, esoteric, or unpractical to your personality's logical, insecure way of seeing, I hope you'll not discard them as clichés. If you don't understand them or even if you find yourself resisting or disagreeing with them, just notice the resistance; and instead of rejecting them, place them on a mental shelf labeled "awaiting greater clarity."

These quotes, although attributed to specific authors, are really just those authors' seeing of true reality beyond illusions. Once you begin piercing through the same veil of illusion, you will see the same way and you will feel like you could just as easily have written very similar things, because they are really just descriptions of reality undistorted by illusion. Think of these quotes as previews to your own way of seeing as you begin to clear away all the accumulated illusions and clean the chakra windows of your soul. For now, use them as corrective lenses. When you notice yourself getting upset by how life is appearing to you, try them on. Becoming upset is actually a message that what you're seeing as real is an illusion. I imagine even the authors of these quotes still had (or have) times when they needed the help of corrective lenses themselves. That's the nature of the human experience for now; the illusions are constantly trying to close in around us, and the moment we believe them, they look very real to us.

PART I
Overview and Personal Story

1

A QUICK OVERVIEW OF THE SPIRAL UP YOGA SYSTEM

Spiral Up Yoga is a simple, practical, yoga-based daily self-care system for body, mind, and soul. The system is chakra based and tied to the days of the week as follows:

- Monday is First Chakra day

- Tuesday is Second Chakra day

- Wednesday is Third Chakra day

- Thursday is Fourth Chakra day

- Friday is Fifth Chakra day

- Saturday is Sixth Chakra day

- Sunday is Seventh Chakra day

The system has only one simple rule:

Do something each day, no matter how small, to open and strengthen that day's chakra.

During each week I will have done something to strengthen all seven chakras, and this complete cycle is repeated every week. Each week becomes one cycle in an ever-expanding spiral – hence the name Spiral Up Yoga.

The practice takes just a few minutes a day and can be done without an instructor anywhere I am, and at any time of the day. I don't even have to change my clothes or unroll my yoga mat to do it. The success of the system is based on the powerful principle behind all growth and progress: small and simple actions repeated consistently over time lead to lasting transformation. Each day I do at least one thing designed to strengthen that day's chakra. Some days I'll do only one thing that takes just a minute; some days I'll do multiple things and may spend ten to fifteen minutes total. But on average, all I need is five minutes a day.

The tools that I use to strengthen that day's chakra may include specific yoga positions, specific sounds I make with my own voice, specific breath work, specific tuning fork vibrations, smelling specifically designed essential oils, focusing on specific mindsets to elicit specific emotions, or various other simple little things – all of which I will teach you in this book.

Spiral Up Yoga doesn't replace other forms of exercise. I still run, bike, swim, or do long yoga sets at times, but they are not consistent, daily practices. What Spiral Up Yoga has become for me is a daily foundation practice, so that even on days when I do nothing else, I know I have still done something that day to strengthen that day's chakra.

Spiral Up Yoga is not a rigid system that you must conform to. It is not a goal-based system where you are trying to get to a certain weight or a certain level. It is not a system of escalating commitment that requires more time or greater commitment as you progress. It is completely customizable. People can experiment and create their own ways of doing it that best fit their lives. Over time, as their situations change, they can evolve and alter their own ways of doing it. Spiral Up Yoga works no matter your age or level of experience with yoga, and it is a lifelong practice. With its unforgettably simple structure and its unlimited ways of personalizing, there is no end to the ways you can create your own practice and the depth to which you can take it.

② HOW I CAME TO CREATE SPIRAL UP YOGA

Before I discovered the benefits of yoga myself, I had heard of it, but I had written it off as a new-age, mostly feminine form of exercise that just wasn't my style. I preferred more manly forms like weight lifting and biking and running. As I got into my thirties, my body began to experience some breakdowns. One morning in 2005, as I was just getting out of bed, I felt a tremendous pain in my lower back that shot through my whole body. At first I thought I might have pulled a muscle, but the pain stayed and began to shoot down my left leg. Then I noticed numbness in my left foot. My doctor put me on pain medication and muscle relaxants and ordered an MRI. The MRI revealed that I had herniated the L4-L5 disc in my lower spine. The disc was pressing against my sciatic nerve on the left side, which was causing the numbness in my left leg. It took almost six months before I was back to normal. But my normal had become a state of being that was far below what was actually available to me. I didn't see it that way at the time, but now I do.

That experience was a wake-up call for me. I now saw that despite exercising fairly regularly, my body had become unbalanced and inflexible. The lower-back injury was just a result of the underlying imbalance and tension in my body. I began to notice how inflexible I had become. I could not bend over and touch my toes while keeping my knees straight. I could maybe reach the mid-point of my shins (just to show you that you can recover lost flexibility, I can now put my palms flat on the floor). I knew this was not the way my body was naturally designed to be. I had allowed it to become stiff and inflexible through my actions and inaction.

Still, the thought of yoga didn't really occur to me at that point. I tried some stretching exercises and started walking and then jogging, slowly getting back into my old routines, but I knew at some level that if I didn't change something, it was just a matter of time before I injured myself again. I also wanted to find a physical practice that worked on more than a physical level – something that worked on body, mind, and soul. I went exploring for something new. I got curious about marital arts first.

I reasoned that martial arts had been around for thousands of years in the Asian cultures, and the thought of becoming a trained martial artist appealed to my masculine ego. I tried a few classes, but it seemed like it really just focused mostly on kicking and punching and sparring, and I didn't see it as the holistic body/mind/soul practice I was looking for and that I could sustain as a lifelong practice. I'm not saying that some forms of martial arts can't do that, but my experience of the commercial establishments in my area didn't feel right for me.

I DISCOVER DAHN YOGA

Then one day I saw a brochure in a store for a form of yoga called Dahn yoga. It was of Korean origin, and it claimed to work on body, mind, and soul all at the same time. It also had its own version of martial arts called DahnMuDo. I was intrigued enough by the brochure to go to the place and check it out. I went to a free class as a walk-in to see what it was all about. I met the local master, Alex Lee, and was struck by his presence. His body was lean, strong, flexible, and agile. His demeanor was calm and assured, his eyes were bright and friendly, and I could tell he was a spiritually evolved person I could learn from on many levels.

I enrolled and began going to sessions at five-thirty a.m. on Tuesdays and Thursdays. One of the first things I realized was just how stiff and inflexible my body had become. I also began to see how the inflexibility of my body seemed to be a mirror of the inflexibility of my mind. Over time, as I began to increase in the flexibility of my body, I noticed that my thinking became more flexible too. This manifested itself in less judgment and more compassion toward others and myself, and a greater openness to new ideas and ways of being.

During the time I trained there, I was exposed to many ideas and ways of seeing life that were new to me. After about two years of fairly consistent practice with Master Lee, I had learned a lot, and my body and mind had become much more flexible and agile. I felt more balanced and grounded, more energetic, and more calm-minded, peaceful, and loving. I had also experienced actually feeling my energy body and had been educated in understanding the chakra and meridian system of the energy body. There were frequent moments of experiencing my connection to all others and to infinite intelligence, or cosmic energy, as Master Lee would refer to it.

But by this time, I was beginning to see that the Dahn yoga system, as wonderful as it was, was turning into too much of a time commitment. It also began to seem a bit like a religion or a club. I held no judgment against their systems; in fact, if anything I judged them as highly beneficial. But I wanted to explore other forms of yoga, and I was finding that the time commitment was not sustainable for me.

I EXPLORE OTHER FORMS OF YOGA

So I began exploring other forms of yoga. I next tried Bikram yoga, which is the "hot" yoga where they heat the room up to one hundred degrees and you perform a regimented set of twenty-six asanas (yoga positions) that takes ninety minutes to complete. It was very physically demanding and I enjoyed the challenge of it, but once again the time commitment proved unsustainable for me.

Next I tried other forms of more traditional yoga like Ashtanga, Vinyasa, and Hatha. I enjoyed these as well, but once again found that the time required to change clothes, drive to class, and return home was often ninety minutes to two hours each time – not exactly something I could do on a daily basis.

In my quest to make a daily yoga practice more practical and sustainable, I decided to try buying some DVDs and doing yoga in front of my TV screen, directed by the instructor on the DVD. Among the various DVDs I tried, I really took a liking to a form called Kundalini yoga. I was able to eliminate the commute to class and also find yoga sets that only took twenty to thirty minutes but still left me feeling great.

But even with the shorter time commitment, I still found that days and sometimes weeks would slip by without practicing. Then I would get into it for a while, only to see it wane as life got busy or my other forms of exercise took up my available time.

I began to create my own little mini-sets that I could do in just a few minutes. I discovered that even just a few minutes shortly after arising in the morning or right before going to bed at night gave me many of the same body, mind, and soul benefits that the much longer sets did.

THE ENERGY BODY

During these years of practicing various forms of yoga, I also became fascinated with understanding more about the energy body. I did online research and read many books about the topic. I learned a lot more about the chakras and meridians and how they could be affected by all sorts of things – not just by doing the physical yoga asanas (positions). I learned that in addition to the physical asanas, the chakras of the energy body could be strengthened through color, sound, vibration, smell, breath work, emotion, mindset, and even various activities.

I also learned more about how interconnected the physical body and organs are with the energy body and how chronic neglect of the energy body would inevitably manifest itself in a chronic condition in the physical body. There also appeared to be a strong connection between a chronic condition in the physical body and a specific chakra that supported that organ or system. I decided that I wanted to design a simple self-care practice that helped me keep my energy body in good shape as a preventative effort to stay healthier now and in the future.

I began experimenting with other chakra-strengthening methods and adding them to my yoga practice. I found that even on days when I didn't fit in any yoga asanas, I could still easily use one of these other methods as a way of opening and strengthening my chakras. But still, I would once again often go days and sometimes weeks without doing any of this. I knew how beneficial it was; I just didn't have a simple enough system yet to keep me consistent.

IT ALL COMES TOGETHER IN A FLASH OF INSPIRATION

And then one day in January 2008, it hit me. There are seven days of the week and seven major chakras. Why not just use that simple fact and design a practice around it? Monday would be First Chakra day, when I would do one or more things that opened and strengthened my First Chakra. On Tuesday I would do the same for my Second Chakra. During the course of one week, I would have done something to stimulate and strengthen all seven chakras, and then I would just repeat that process each week – but with each repetition of the cycle, I would be building cumulatively upon the last and all that came before it, and so it would proceed in what I saw as an upward spiral.

That flash of inspiration was the birth of Spiral Up Yoga. I spent months afterwards cataloging and organizing all my favorite yoga asanas by which chakra they most strengthened. I incorporated other methods of chakra stimulation and strengthening such as toning, mantras, aromatherapy, tuning fork vibration, emotional stimulation, and mindset focus.

The end result was a simple system based on a single, simple rule. There were infinite ways to customize the system. It took only a few minutes a day and was enjoyable to do. I knew I had finally found a self-care practice that was balanced and benefited my body, my mind, and my soul and that I would do it for the rest of my life. Even if I were bedridden, I could do something that day to stimulate and strengthen that day's chakra. It might not be a backward bend, but I could at least do the breath work, sound the tone with my voice, or deeply inhale the specific aromatherapy oil.

THEN IT SITS ON MY BACK BURNER FOR FOUR YEARS

For nearly four years after first having the inspiration to create Spiral Up Yoga, I made it my own foundational practice, tweaking and evolving it. I shared bits and pieces with a few family members, but for the most part I was satisfied just using it as my own private practice. I knew that there were probably lots of other people who would really benefit from learning the Spiral Up Yoga system, but I was engaged in other entrepreneurial endeavors, and I convinced myself it would be too costly and time-consuming to bring this practice to the market.

Then in late 2011 I felt my soul really push me to bring Spiral Up Yoga to others. I started talking to a few people I had met since first developing my system, and before long I knew what I had to do. I had to create a book and a website and do what I could to share Spiral Up Yoga with the world, and I needed to put all the other projects I was involved in on the back burner until I did so. The fact that you are reading this now is proof that I've done that.

PART 2
The Life Coaching Foundation

SELF-CARE: THE FOUNDATION OF PERSONAL GROWTH

Yesterday I was clever, so I wanted to change the world.
Today I am wise, so I am changing myself.
– RUMI

There comes a point in everyone's journey of personal growth where they realize that having a daily self-care practice is an essential foundation for continual growth, health, well-being, and creative inspiration. It is also a source of resilience, strength, perspective, and peace of mind during particularly challenging times when things aren't going the way you might prefer.

By self-care, I mean more than just an exercise program. I mean a daily, sustainable practice that feeds and nourishes body, mind, and soul. Practices that only include one or two of the three elements are good, but not complete. They are usually not sustainable in the long run, because if the body, the mind, or the soul is neglected enough, your whole system becomes unstable, like a three-legged stool with one or more weak legs.

Ask truly joyful, creative, successful people, and you will find that they have developed or adopted their own form of self-care – something that keeps them grounded and connected with their soul and their source, and helps them maintain an energetic and healthy body and mind with which to create and serve.

Having happy relationships, a fulfilling career, an exercise routine and a spiritual
practice are even more important to health than a daily diet.
- JOSHUA ROSENTHAL

SHARPENING THE SAW

ANALOGY
Sharpening the Saw

Steven Covey, in his best-selling book The Seven Habits of Highly Effective People, listed as the seventh habit what he called "sharpening the saw." He used the analogy of cutting down trees with a saw and compared two different strategies. The first strategy was to never take the time to sharpen the saw because it took valuable time away from cutting down trees. As the saw got duller and duller, the amount of energy and time required to cut down trees increased. The other strategy was to take time away from cutting down trees to sharpen the saw so that it cut with the least amount of effort required for the job. He compared the sharpening of the saw to renewing yourself physically, mentally, and spiritually – in other words, to having a good self-care practice.

STAYING CONNECTED TO THE VINE

A good self-care practice is what keeps me connected to the vine of life so that energy, wisdom, and intelligence can flow through me from a deeper source than my own personality. Think of a grape vine that is connected to its roots. It draws nourishment and life from being connected. The moment the vine becomes severed from the roots is the moment that the withering process begins. The same is true for me (and you). I draw my energy, my health, my creativity, my wisdom and knowledge not from myself alone, but from maintaining my connection with my source. When I allow myself to become disconnected, the withering process begins. It doesn't matter how long I've been connected to my source in the past; the moment I disconnect, the withering process begins. Fortunately, unlike a grape vine that has been disconnected from its source, I can always reconnect myself to my source – and the moment I do that, no matter how long I've been disconnected, the re-enlivening process begins.

> *There are dead branches and live branches full of sap.*
> *The sun brings flowers and fruit from one and more withering to the other.*
> – RUMI

ANALOGY
Staying Connected to the Vine

A NEW WAY OF SEEING JUSTICE & MERCY

This, to me, is one way to understand what the Bible refers to as the law of justice and the law of mercy. The law of justice is simply this: the moment I disconnect myself from my source, I begin to wither. It's not personal; it's not like I've been singled out by a vengeful God to be punished. Nothing of the sort. I've just allowed myself to become disconnected, and the natural consequence when we allow ourselves to disconnect is that we begin to wither. The source of energy, health, wisdom, and creativity is not actually self-contained within us; rather, it flows through us.

DISTINCTION
A New Way of Seeing Justice & Mercy

The law of mercy is simply this: no matter how long I've managed to stay disconnected, the moment I reconnect, the re-enlivening process begins and I receive a new flow of energy, health, wisdom, and creativity. The law of mercy is also impersonal in that it doesn't keep score and it never blacklists me. It doesn't say, "Well, you've had enough chances and you keep blowing them, so no more flow of good stuff for you this time." No. If I've disconnected and reconnected myself a thousand times, on the thousand and first time I reconnect, the flow is reestablished and begins to grow and enliven me.

This is why I have a saying I love to use, which is this:

"If life were fair, I'd be much worse off."

Think about that for a moment. In what ways are you better off because life isn't fair, but rather merciful? Life is, in fact, better than fair; it is merciful. How many chances does

Life give you to learn what you're here to learn? As many as you're willing to allow; and then some! How fair is that?

WHAT IS YOUR SELF-CARE PRACTICE?

So what is your self-care practice? How consistent are you in keeping your saw sharp and reconnecting to the vine? Does your practice include something that sharpens your body, your mind, and your soul on a regular basis and keeps you connected to the vine? How much time do you give it on a daily or weekly basis?

You don't need to give a lot of time to it. In fact, keeping it small and simple actually proves to be a more powerful way than trying to make big breakthroughs with major bursts of energy or taking on practices that require large time commitments or lots of discipline and willpower. I can only speak for myself, but anything that requires more than about five minutes a day I have found to be unsustainable as a daily practice over the long run.

Fierce winds do not blow all morning;
A downpour of rain does not last the day.
Who does this? Heaven and earth.
But these are exaggerated, forced effects,
And that is why they cannot be sustained.
If heaven and earth cannot sustain a forced action,
How much less is man able to do so?
- LAO TZU

THE POWER OF SMALL AND SIMPLE REPEATED CONSISTENTLY OVER TIME

Throughout my life, I've experimented with lots of different types of self-care practices, including:

- Training for and running a marathon

- Biking regimens

- Swimming regimens

- Weight lifting regimens

- Detoxing protocols

- Diet protocols

- Nutritional supplement protocols

- Meditation practices

- Journaling and free-writing practices

- Reading and studying sacred texts

I'm sure I've benefited from them all, but most of these attempts proved (for me, anyway) to be unsustainable after a while. I usually started them with great gusto and a firm resolve to stick with it, but eventually I would get too busy, lose interest, or try something new. I still do some of these things, but not on a daily basis. The self-care practices I've benefited the most from are the ones that I stick with most consistently and over the long term. There is a principle at play here that is evident throughout nature as well. The principle is that small, simple actions repeated consistently over time lead to major growth and lasting transformation. By this principle, water can cut through solid stone.

Moderation, simplicity and consistency over intensity. I created Spiral Up Yoga based on this principle. The daily practice is small and simple, taking only five minutes. Each week you complete a full cycle, evolving it and customizing it to your situation as you go.

> *Most of us are vigilant when making big decisions, but less so when dealing with little ones. We forget the cumulative effect of all those missed "little" opportunities. It is precisely on those thousand little occasions, and over a period of time, that the mind is taught to be calm and kind – not instantaneously or by great leaps. In the ordinary choices of every day we begin to change the direction of our lives.*
> – EKNATH EASWAREN

WHY SPIRAL UP YOGA IS A SUSTAINABLE, LIFELONG SELF-CARE PRACTICE

I've found that when it comes to my own self-care, there are two primary factors that seem to determine how long I can sustain a particular practice. Assuming that I experience the self-care practice as beneficial to my body, mind, or soul, the two factors that determine how long I sustain that practice are:

1. How much of a time commitment it requires. Generally, the more time required, the shorter the amount of time I am able to sustain it.

2. How much I actually enjoy the process. Obviously, the more I enjoy the actual process, the more I will tend to do it and the longer I will tend to sustain it. I'm more likely to enjoy practices that give me quick, beneficial results than I am to enjoy practices where the major benefits are only experienced way down the road.

Check this against your own experience. Do you agree?

Even if I enjoy and benefit from a particular practice, if it takes too much time, life just gets in the way too often and despite my best intentions, I find I'm not able to sustain it for very long. Conversely, if something doesn't take a lot of time, but I don't get an intrinsic reward directly from taking the action, I won't tend to sustain that either, even if the future benefits are desirable.

Spiral Up Yoga is a sustainable, lifelong self-care practice because it meets both of the criteria I've listed above.

1. It doesn't demand a lot of time – it only takes about five minutes a day.

2. It provides a direct intrinsic reward every time you practice it, benefitting body, mind, and soul at the same time.

You actually feel in your body a relaxing and an energizing at the same time. You begin to feel a little less stiff and a little looser in your joints and muscles as tension that has been stored there is released. You actually feel your mind get a little calmer and feel more peace in your heart as your stressed and overactive thinking quiets down for a while. You begin to experience the other mode of thought – the flow mode where insight, wisdom, and creativity come from. You actually feel the innate qualities of your soul begin to shine forth a little brighter as the heavy thinking and emotional cloud cover dissipates.

You must be the kind of man who can get things done. But to get things done, you must love the doing, not the secondary consequences.
- AYN RAND

THE THREE I'S WITHIN I

As I explained in the Introduction to this book, Spiral Up Yoga is much more than just another yoga program. Spiral Up Yoga is ultimately about your personal transformation at the simultaneous levels of body, mind, and soul. But what does that really mean – body, mind, and soul? It's a phrase that gets used often without really being clear on what it means. I also use the phrase to describe how Spiral Up Yoga impacts you, so I thought I'd also explain what I mean by the phrase.

Among all the many distinctions I've realized so far, the most foundational is the distinction that I call "The Three I's Within I." When I refer to myself, I use the word "I," but there is so much wrapped up within "I" that it can be really confusing to understand "I" if I'm not clear on who "I" really am. When I say "I," there are actually three separate but also overlapping "I"s, which I distinguish by the names:

1.   Body (Physical Self)

2.   Personality (Apparent Self)

3.   Soul (Essential Self)

In this distinction, I have deliberately chosen the word personality in place of mind. The reason is because the personality is primarily how we experience mind. Mind itself is impossible to accurately define, but I'll do my best by saying that mind is the infinite realm in which all thoughts exist.

Of the infinite amount of thoughts that exist, all of them can be categorized into two categories: 1) true and self-evident and 2) false and illusory. Our personality is basically a subset of thoughts that exist within mind; thoughts that have been woven together about who we are and what we're capable of and how we relate to each other and to all of life. My personality is something that was invented by my childhood perception of what would make me safe. So is yours. Most (maybe even all) of the thoughts that make up your personality are not original or self-generated, but rather pre-existing, recycled thoughts that have been around since the beginning of time. Most, if not all, of the thoughts that make up your personality are also of the false and illusory type.

My intent is to create greater clarity, not greater confusion, and I realize I run the risk of creating greater confusion by trying to address such a huge topic in so few words. A true realization of the nature of mind and personality cannot really be had through words, anyway; it can only be individually experienced and known directly through what some Zen masters call a happy accident. This means it just happens at some point in the course of each individual's evolutionary unfolding, and cannot be systemized and duplicated. I believe that is true, but I also believe that the more clear we can be intellectually about this distinction of the three I's, the more we are likely to be prone to a happy accident.

The more clear I am about my Three I's, their nature and their ways of interacting, the more easily I notice which of my "I's" is asserting itself most at any given moment. All three are always present, but the relative balance of the three is dynamic and constantly changing. The practice of yoga is the best practice of which I am aware to consistently bring all three into alignment and unity with each other.

Let us briefly explore the basic nature of each of the three "I's." What follows is a highly distilled version of my current level of clarity around these topics. Please don't take them as absolute and unquestionable truths, but run them against your own personal experience of life.

BODY: THE PHYSICAL SELF

The body is the physical self. It is an amazing physical vehicle through which both the personality and the soul can operate in this physical dimension. The body has its own innate intelligence (part of mind), which is operating all the time. I cut my finger and my body knows how to heal the wound; and it goes about doing it on its own. It doesn't need or ask for my permission, it just knows what to do and does it. When I eat or drink, my body knows what to do with what I feed it. My cells divide and multiply, my hair grows, my heart pumps, my diaphragm expands and contracts to bring in the energy and air that exist all around me. There are literally trillions of highly interrelated and amazingly sophisticated activities happening every second that are being monitored and regulated by my body, all with the purpose of maintaining the best possible balance to sustain the life of the body.

The nature of my body is to maintain balance and sustain life, and eventually to reproduce physical life. The body is also temporary in nature. It creates itself from two microscopic cells that contain within them all the intelligence necessary to assemble from the appropriate environment all the raw materials needed to create and sustain a body. The raw materials are constantly replaced from the environment as the body grows and ages, and eventually the body either breaks down enough or is damaged enough that it ceases to be a viable physical vehicle for the personality and the soul, and we call that death. After death, the body returns all its current store of raw materials to the environment from which it drew them.

The body is both separate and one. It is a separate physical vehicle, but at the same time is one with all other bodies, as they all draw upon the same environment for physical existence and the same intelligence of Life that orchestrates the process of physical life.

This body is not me. It is the house in which I live. If you say that I am so many inches tall, or that I weigh such and such number of pounds, I will reply, "You are not describing me. You are talking about my address."
- EKNATH EASWAREN

Man's true self is eternal,
Yet he thinks, I am this body and will soon die.
- LAO TZU

PERSONALITY: THE APPARENT SELF

Personalities don't love - they want something.
- BYRON KATIE

My personality is my "apparent self" because it is whom I have come to think of as "me." It's who I think I am, not who I really am. The word "personality" comes from the root word "persona," and "persona" comes from Latin and means "mask" or "character." What we would call actors today, in Latin would be called personas. The personality is really a construction of many different masks or characters, the totality of which becomes a personality. The personality doesn't exist until early childhood, and by late childhood it is pretty much in place and convinced it is running the show. I know many parents will insist that their children come with pre wired personalities, and as a parent of six children I understand why they would believe that. However, I believe these early differences that clearly exist before the formation of a personality can happen, are really soul traits. I'll get to the soul in the next section.

My personality is a construction of all the beliefs, assumptions and conditioning that it has accepted as true even if most if not all are actually illusory and not true. I experience my personality largely as the voice inside my head that narrates my existence. Sometimes I refer to my personality as "the roommate" because it is almost like another person who shares my body with my soul.

Because my personality is a mental construction, and not "real" like my body and soul, there are certain qualities that are inherent in its nature. Here are a few you might recognize. It is inherently insecure and defensive. It never feels like it is ready, but always "under construction." I like to say it is always "getting ready to get ready." Its essential identity is one of "becoming" but never "being." It is constantly comparing itself to others around it trying to gauge where it stacks up against the competition. It is vigilant and wary of attack from any and all sources. It rehashes past events and keeps alive old hurts. It is frequently anxious and worried about what might happen in the future. It feels lonely and isolated and empty and seeks to fill the emptiness by seeking money, accomplishments, relationships, and pleasant experiences. Essentially the personality is looking for everything that the soul already has in inexhaustible abundance, but it's awareness is focused in the external world.

What is the difference
Between your experience of Existence
And that of a saint?
The saint knows
That the spiritual path
Is a sublime chess game with God
And that the Beloved
Has just made such a fantastic Move
That the saint is now continually
Tripping over Joy
And bursting out in Laughter
And saying "I Surrender!"
Whereas, my dear,
I am afraid you still think
You have a thousand serious moves.
– Hafiz

Some may think that the personality is something to be extinguished if you are to attain "enlightenment." But the personality is an essential part of "I." The personality is the lens through which the soul experiences separateness which is actually something the soul wants to experience and chose to come into this life to experience. The goal here is not to extinguish the personality (which isn't really possible anyway), but to appreciate it and allow it to relax and let the soul and body play a more active role in directing the course of life. The personality really just wants to be appreciated and included. It doesn't want to have to work as hard as it does to feel safe and loved.

Every act of conscious learning requires the willingness to suffer an injury to one's self-esteem. That is why young children, before they are aware of their own self-importance, learn so easily; and why older persons, especially if vain or important, cannot learn at all.
- Dr. Thomas Szasz

Most people live, whether physically, intellectually or morally, in a very restricted circle of their potential being. They make use of a very small portion of their possible consciousness, and of their soul's resources in general, much like a man who, out of his whole bodily organism, should get into a habit of using and moving only his little finger.
– William James

SOUL: THE ESSENTIAL SELF

How do I know the ways of all things at the beginning?
I look inside myself and see what is within me.
- LAO TZU

You are not saintly because an organization says so, but rather because you stay connected to the divinity of your origination. You are not intelligent because of a transcript; you are intelligence itself, which needs no external confirmation. You are not moral because you obey the laws; you are morality itself because you are the same as what you came from.
- WAYNE DYER

To me it is abundantly clear that I have a soul; and this is not just through intellectual understanding or religious teaching, but through direct experiencing of the soul as my essential self. There are many other terms often used as names for what I am calling the soul, such as spirit, essential self, true self, or authentic self.

Here is how I would explain my soul, keeping in mind that any explanation in words is grossly inadequate.

My soul is something that existed prior to my body being assembled and will continue to exist after my body disassembles itself. My soul is immortal in that it cannot cease to exist and to be aware. It exists beyond time and space but also within the time I call my lifetime and the space I call my body.

My soul has its own innate nature that it brings with it into my body. There are many soul qualities that are common among all human beings, because a human being is really a soul being human. Some of the qualities of the soul that are apparent to me include unconditional love, compassion, freedom, service, patience, gratitude, joy, creative expression, and fearless exploring. The soul comes into this physical life on purpose and with certain lessons it is here to learn, or further master, and with already existent strengths and abilities it is here to serve with. When a baby is born, and in early childhood, we can more easily notice the innate soul qualities shining forth more clearly than we can in most adults. This is because the personality has not been fully formed and has not yet taken over control of the baby's awareness. Being around little children can penetrate the personality in adults and resonate at a deep soul level, which is what makes them so enjoyable to be around.

For the most part, the soul operates quietly in the background and waits patiently for the personality to invite it to be a more active partner. Occasionally, the soul will exert itself more obviously, like in moments of existential crisis or near-death experiences, but generally it waits to be invited to take a more active role in everyday decisions. The nature of the soul is pure being. Many of the eastern spiritual practices refer to it as the Self (capitalized), the Witness, or pure awareness.

Every man, woman and child has a soul
And it is the destiny of all,
To see as God sees, to know as God knows
To be as God Is.
- MEISTER ECKHART

WHO IS SPEAKING WHEN I SAY "I"?

Of course much more has and could be said about the body, personality and soul. The main point here is to just begin to recognize the separate but overlapping existence of all three and to begin to notice the nature of each. Then when you say "I," you can further ask one of the most clarity-enhancing questions I know of:

"Who is speaking when I say 'I'?"

When you say, "I am upset at her," which I is upset and why? When you say, "I beat myself up all week long over what I said to her," who is beating up whom? And who did the speaking to her anyway that is the source of regret and shame? When you say, "I'm hungry," which I is hungry? Is it really the body that needs nourishment, or might it be the personality that is feeling anxious or lonely and has learned that eating makes it feel safer for a while? When you say, "I don't know what to do or I need to know what to do," which I are you talking about? The personality or the soul?

The more you inquire into this deeper level of identity, the more apparent it becomes that the personality is desperately trying to fight an unwinnable battle. It is trying to create safety, love, and connection through external means; and therefore even when it temporarily feels safe, loved, and connected, it is constantly worried that something external will threaten that – and with good reason, because it's true. Life is kind that way; always trying to help the personality learn that everything it tries to substitute for the soul will not allow it to feel secure because it is an illusion of security only, not true security. The personality may not see it as kind at the time, but eventually it comes to see the kindness.

CAR, DRIVER & PASSENGER

I was driving my car one day and reflecting on this idea of the three I's when it hit me that driving my car was actually a great analogy to understand the three I's. My body is like the car. It is the vehicle that allows me to get around and operate within this physical dimension. It has its own built-in intelligence, but without a driver, it's powerless to do anything. So who is the driver in this analogy? Well, most of the time it is my personality who is

ANALOGY
Car, Driver, Passenger

20

really in the driver's seat, and my soul is usually in the passenger seat – or more likely in the back seat, or maybe even shoved back in the trunk!

I see one of life's basic purposes is to help us learn how to invite the soul to take a more active role in driving the car – to at least be the navigator in the passenger seat and maybe even take stints at driving the car so the personality can relax and rest a bit. Eventually, when the personality has learned to trust and allow and not need to be in charge, the soul can return to its rightful role as the primary driver and the personality can then enjoy a much more interesting journey free of fear and anxiety and the constant need to control.

> *There is a Beautiful Creature*
> *Living in a hole you have dug.*
> *I have fallen in love with Someone*
> *Who hides inside you.*
> *We should talk about this problem–*
> *Otherwise,*
> *I will never leave you alone.*
> *– HAFIZ*

THE LANGUAGES OF PERSONALITY, BODY AND SOUL

When it comes to what drives our actions to do anything, including to create a daily self-care practice for body, mind (personality), and soul, it's useful to see where the prompt to act, or to not act, is coming from. It's especially useful to understand this when you are exploring making a change to your current routines and venturing outside your safety zones, which is exactly what I'm inviting you to do by reading this book and experimenting with Spiral Up Yoga.

Now that we have established the foundational distinction of the body, personality, and soul, let's see how this can help us be clearer on which of these three parts of self is motivating our action or inaction. Since we know that the personality is usually in the driver's seat, it's a good bet that the motivation to act or not act is most likely coming from the personality. There are exceptions, but we'll get to those soon.

MOTIVATION & FEAR: THE LANGUAGE OF THE PERSONALITY

Because it is constructed almost entirely of illusory thoughts, the personality is generally coming from a place of insecurity. The personality is motivated from a belief that it is never enough and always needs to improve itself so it can perceive itself as worthy and safe and secure; and only then it can relax. Counterbalancing this tendency to seek for constant improvement is an equally strong tendency to not venture far from the known; to stay within the bounds that it thinks represents the best chance for safety. So if taking on a new practice involves venturing into the unknown, even if there appears to be some self-improvement in it for the personality, there will often be a tug-of-war going on within the personality that will make sustained action difficult and usually end up in a confusing soup of self-justification and self-condemnation.

But who is doing the self-justifying and who is doing the self-condemning? The personality is justifying itself and condemning itself. The body and soul are basically on the sidelines watching in patient amusement and compassion.

For some reason, it is very difficult for us to accept our divine nature. This has always puzzled me. We pay money for books about how destructive we are. We stand in line to see movies that emphasize our capacity for making trouble. Then, when Jesus comes to tell us that the kingdom of heaven is within us, we say, "There must be some mistake." It is to convince us that our real Self is always pure and eternal that men and women of God keep arising among us. More than anything, we need to hear their good news that the source of all joy and security is right within.
— EKNATH EASWAREN

APPETITES & SYMPTOMS: THE LANGUAGE OF THE BODY

To maintain balance and sustain life, the body is coming from a place of innate well-being and intelligence. It will prompt us to action or inaction only based on helping it to receive the basic physical and energetic inputs it needs to do its job. When it is not getting what it needs to perform its job of balancing and sustaining, or when it is being given too much of what harms it, the body will speak up in the form of a physical symptom. Pain, aches, fever, tiredness, thirst, hunger, and diseases are examples we've all experienced. These symptoms are really the language of the body. They are gifts, trying to recapture a bit of attention away from the personality. If the personality ignores the symptom-based communication of the body for long enough, the body will exert itself and create a situation that the personality cannot ignore any longer, like a serious disease or injury, or a debilitating depression or migraine.

Appetite is something that is really the body's to control, but it often gets usurped by the personality. Severe imbalances in appetite such as anorexia or obesity are personality disorders, not body disorders. In these cases the body is just the victim, doing its very best to deal with the extreme imbalance of inputs given to it by the personality.

Consider the body a robe you wear. When you meet someone you love, do you kiss their clothes? Search out who's inside.
– RUMI

EXPRESSION & INSPIRATION: THE LANGUAGE OF THE SOUL

The soul is always coming from a place of expressing its innate nature, which is joy, service, love, freedom, belonging, creation, and evolving (to name just a few of its innate qualities). The soul is here to experience life through the lens of a personality and body in a physical dimension. Its desire is to experience life fully from this perspective and to guide the personality into learning how to release its need for control and allow the soul to take a more active role in living. The soul also comes with specific purposes or callings that it is here to contribute to others. It will prompt and prod the personality to move in that direction through what we sometimes call the desire of the heart. The soul is patient and resourceful. While it may be able to see that going down one road might be better for it than going down another, it will usually leave the decision up to the personality. It knows that whatever road the personality chooses, the soul will be perfectly able to use whatever comes down that road to help the personality learn what it needs to learn – which is always more allowing, more releasing, more trusting.

THE SIX POWERS

With this understanding of the basic nature of the personality, body, and soul, let's now quickly look at six powers that prompt us into action or inaction, and how each one operates. The six powers I speak of are as follows:

1. Illusion Power

2. Will Power

3. Want Power

4. Still Power

5. Coach Power

6. Tribe Power

ILLUSION POWER

While illusion power can appear very powerful, it is ultimately impotent. It is powerful when we lend to it the power of our belief, and it becomes impotent when we withdraw the power of our belief. When we believe an illusion, that illusion will have tremendous power over us, limiting our perception to what the illusion allows us to see.

The personality is largely formed of illusions that borrow their power from our belief in them. So long as we believe in and perceive the illusions to be real, we live as though they are and so the net effect is that to us, they are real. There are collective illusions that entire societies and multiple generations support with their belief, and then there are individualized illusions that make up each of our own personal hells that we believe are unique to us (even though they are really generic and recycled and commonplace). For example, for many generations it was commonly believed that the world was flat and revolved around the sun. That illusion had great power so long as it was collectively believed. It kept people from venturing too far away for fear of falling off the edge of the world. It took a few misfits who stopped lending their belief to the illusion for that illusion to become impotent for them, and eventually for everyone. The impotence of the belief that the world is flat seems so obvious to us today, but there are many more illusions to which we still lend our belief, collectively or individually; and as a result they still have great power over us – mostly the power to limit us from pressing beyond them.

I jump the fence of illusion, and end up in Heaven.
- DREAMING-BEAR, BARAKA KANAAN

ANALOGY
Rubber Bands and Will Power

WILL POWER AND MOTIVATION

Next to illusion power, will power is a favorite tool of the personality. Although will power is the most often spoken of in the realm of action and achievement, it is actually the least powerful one of the six. Will power is basically an override – a forcing of action in one direction while there is a strong counter force pulling in the opposite direction. This is like trying to move forward while your arms and legs are tied to thick rubber bands secured to a fixed beam. Progress can be forced, but only with the expenditure of extreme and often futile effort. For example, if the personality is more comfortable sleeping in, rarely exercising, and eating whatever it wants whenever it wants, but at the same time the personality sees that this is resulting in it becoming more insecure, not less, it will often marshal up some will power to override the inertia of staying within its comfort zone. With that will-power it will get itself to start an exercise or diet program and to say "no" to the second helping of food or dessert. But without understanding the pull of those attached rubber bands pulling in the opposite direction, will power is almost always eventually overpowered by stronger illusion powered beliefs of the personality that are being threatened by the will power-induced actions.

Your belief will trump your motivation every time.
– MANDY EVANS

Even if the personality sees that having a good self-care practice would be beneficial, if developing a self-care practice takes a lot of time and energy and only pays off way down the road, the personality might be able to use will power to force itself to begin a new practice and stick with it for a little while. It may be able to discipline itself to get up at five a.m. and run in the cold in order to put in the required number of miles to be ready for a race. It may be able to remind itself of the bigger picture and what's at stake by suffering through the hard work. But ultimately it's not sustainable for very long because by its nature, will power consumes more energy than it creates.

I've had clients and friends tell me that they really want to have a good self-care practice, but they just can't seem to motivate themselves to stick with anything long enough for it to make much of a difference. In response, I'll say something like, "I've found that I only have to motivate myself to do something that I don't really want to do. So it only means you haven't yet found something that you really want to do – something that gives you an intrinsic reward every time you do it. Just keep trying things until you find it, and then you won't need to motivate yourself so much. Motivating yourself is exhausting."

Motivation is about getting me to do something I (my personality) thinks I should do, but doesn't really want to do, as evidenced by the observable fact that I'm not doing it. And how do I motivate myself to do something I don't really want to do? It usually takes the form of shame or fear. I may imagine my life being so much better in some way if only I can shame myself enough to do what I'm not doing, because that's what I would do if I were really a good person or if I really wanted to be successful. The other way is through fear. I imagine my life being so much worse in some way unless I motivate myself to do what I'm not doing.

If I am feeling *pushed* to do something that I believe I *should* do, while also feeling resistance to doing it, that is a clear sign that I'm dealing with will power and personality. But because they are too exhausting and soul-sapping, the actions that I (my personality) take out of shame or fear are just not sustainable in the long run.

WANT POWER

Where will power is a fear based push to take action, want power is a love based pull to allow greater expression of the soul. Want power is a natural extension of a pure desire. I take actions because I really want to take them – not for some future reward, but because I enjoy the process of taking the action itself and find intrinsic reward for my body, my personality and my soul, every time I take it. Want power creates energy rather than consuming it. I have more energy after taking an action powered by want power, not less. For example, this book is being written by want power. It's something I really have a strong desire to do and I love the actual process of doing it. I have more energy after a long writing session than I began with. I've learned I can't write late at night because I'm so energized that I can't go to sleep for a long time.

Want power is behind all excellence and mastery in any field of endeavor. The best basketball players are the ones who get intrinsic rewards out of practicing drills and foul shots in solitude, not just out of the thrill of playing for the crowd. The most masterful musicians are the ones who get intrinsic rewards out of practicing scales and arpeggios. The best sales people are the ones who find intrinsic rewards in the actual process of engaging in conversations with prospects and connecting with their wants and needs and finding creative ways to serve them.

STILL POWER

Still power is the power that comes from stilling the active mind (the personality's insecure chatter) and listening to the innate wisdom of the body and the soul. To better understand how still power works, I find this analogy very helpful. Imagine a pool of water. When it's still you can see messages written at the bottom. These messages are coming from your body and soul and represent wisdom, insight and answers to your questions. But you can only see these messages when the water is still. When the water is whipped up by the wind

DISTINCTION
Push vs. Pull Actions

ANALOGY
Pool of Water with Messages on Bottom

or by children splashing in the pool, the messages can't be seen. They don't disappear; they just can't be seen while the water is agitated.

The personality is rarely still enough to access still power, so it resorts to will power instead in an endless and exhausting tug-of-war with itself and its own insecurities. Ironically, in its need to know and do and control, the personality creates the very agitation that prevents it from seeing the guidance and answers that it is seeking.

The muddiest water clears as it is stilled.
And out of that stillness life arises.
- Lao Tzu

As the insecure needs of the personality are sifted out and seen through, and it becomes clear what the soul really desires, still power will often lead to the more powerful want power. That clarity may come in the form of a specific direction to take or not take, or it may come in the form of a peace of mind that you don't really need to know the answers to all your questions right now; that it's actually better that way and to just relax and allow and stay open to what comes next while keeping your attention rooted in gratitude for what is now.

Be still and know that I am God
- Psalms 46:10

The reason this book exists is because during a moment of still power for me, it became really clear that the time was right for me to create a physical product that I could share with the world that was based around my own self-care practice. I had been practicing and evolving Spiral Up Yoga as my own self-care practice for nearly four years. I (my personality) had convinced itself that no one else would really care that much about this, or even if some would, it wouldn't be enough to justify the huge cost involved in creating everything that would need to be created, and then promoting it and managing it. It made no logical sense to add all that work into my already full schedule, and the chances of it paying off financially were slim, and even if it did succeed, did I really want to be known as the yoga guy?

These and other insecure thoughts of my personality kept me from doing anything about it for several years. There was always something deeper tugging at me to not listen to all that and share this with the world. It wasn't until I was able to really get still and listen that it became clear to me that it was time to make this happen and a deep desire to do it was unleashed (want power). But even then, my personality still came up with lots of arguments against doing it, at least for now, maybe later. But no matter how many arguments my personality came up with, the still power clarity and the resulting want power could no longer be ignored and I knew I had to do something about it regardless of the outcome.

Activity conquers cold; Inactivity conquers heat.
Stillness and tranquility set things in order in the Universe.
- LAO TZU

Spiral Up Yoga is a great way to do a little something every day to increase your still power. Everything about yoga assists you at quieting the chatter of the personality and bringing your awareness and attention into the present moment and into the physical body and into the very breath you are breathing. It's like a daily stilling and settling of the agitation in the pool of your mind. Creating a self-care practice that builds your still power is of tremendous value and will be a lifelong source of strength and clarity for you regardless of what comes your way.

The last two powers for creating change are extremely powerful but they cannot be accessed alone, as an individual, no matter how much still power, want power or will power you have. They are catalysts to developing greater personal power as well.

COACH POWER

I call the first one "coach power." A good coach who has a lot of still power themselves, can help you increase your own still power and then support you in seeing through the insecure fear power of the personality's illusions as you begin taking actions inspired by the soul's want power.

I have been able to experience coach power from both sides of the equation – both as a client being coached and as a coach working with clients. Even though I knew I had to do something about getting Spiral Up Yoga out into the world, it wasn't until I sat down with my colleague, friend, and master coach Steve Chandler (who wrote the foreword to this book) and shared with him my thoughts about Spiral Up Yoga that I finally made the internal commitment to get it done and "ship it" (get it out of my head and into the hands of others). I highly recommend making the choice to access the power of coach power, but you'll most likely have to disregard your personality's contesting that you don't need it. The personality sees coaching as a threat to its self-image and an admission that it's not good enough and can't do it all on its own. The body and the soul have no problem what-soever with adding coach power to your life because they see it for what it is – a powerful ally to the body and soul. They know that coach power will help the personality get out of its own way and open itself up to a greater perspective than it would have ever allowed on its own.

If there comes a time in your life when you feel the prompting of your soul, in a moment of still power, to explore what coach power can do for you, I encourage you to follow that prompt. Any money you invest in coaching is really investing in your most valu-able assets – you and your greater clarity. It will pay off in so many ways that include, but completely transcend, financial returns. I offer some coaching programs that help people really extend the transformation that Spiral Up Yoga helps you make. If that calls to you, you can learn more about those on our website.

TRIBE POWER

The second one I call "tribe power," and that is the power that comes from associating yourself with a tribe of people who share your intentions and values and can support and encourage each other. It used to be that your tribe was determined by things outside your control – where you were born, the religion of your parents, the language you spoke, the place you went to school, or the place you worked at. But with the miracles of communications technology today, we can choose to join various tribes whose goals and purposes are aligned with ours, and we can communicate in real time with people from all over the world with whom we share something in common. All the old boundaries that determined our tribe affiliations have largely disappeared, and we can join ourselves with others to whom we would otherwise never have been connected.

If you feel like you'd like to support and be supported by a tribe of people from all over the world who are practicing their own version of Spiral Up Yoga, you can easily join that tribe (for free) at our website.

7

THE TWO MODES OF THINKING

· ·

What I am about to explain in this section is something which, when you really get it, will completely transform your experience of life. I'm not asking you to trust me; I'm asking you to test it for yourself and develop your own trust. This topic alone is worthy of an entire book and training course. In my life and leadership coaching, I do in fact spend a lot of time helping my clients to really see how they use their two modes of thought on a moment-by-moment basis to create their personal experiences of life. For the purposes of this book, I can't go into a lot of depth about it, but I will lay out the basics. Having a basic understanding of your two modes of thought will help you understand at a deeper level what a daily practice of yoga can do for your experience of life.

On the surface, you may think that this doesn't have much to do with yoga. But let me remind you of my definition of yoga.

Anything that helps me bring my body, mind, and soul into greater alignment and unity with each other and with their source is yoga.

There are two modes of thinking that you (and all human beings) experience throughout your life (your waking life, anyway; there are other modes that occur during sleep). These two modes are:

1. Reactive/Directive mode. When it is being misused, which is often, I call this the churn mode.

2. Receptive/Reflective mode, which I like to call the flow mode.

Both modes are important and useful for different situations. It is like a yin/yang balance. Ideally you move back and forth between them and use the mode most appropriate for the situation at hand. I say ideally because most people (myself included) often get stuck in the reactive/directive mode of thinking, which I call churn mode because that is what it feels like. To our great detriment, we spend almost all of our waking time in that state. Practicing yoga is one of the most powerful and simple ways of getting out of churn mode and into receptive/flow mode, which is going to serve you well.

REACTIVE/DIRECTIVE MODE AND CHURNING

Reactive/Directive mode is sometimes called left-brain mode. It is the reactive, processing, analytical mode of thinking and also the mode of thinking that gives directions for taking action. It resembles a computer processor in many ways. It takes information that it has stored and uses it to try to solve problems. It is very effective in certain situations, such as when all the variables are known (or at least believed to be known), or there is only one unknown variable that can be solved for. Reactive thought mode is what allows us to learn something and then repeat it without having to relearn it over and over again. It allows us to learn language and math. It allows us to learn to drive a car, find our way to work and back home again, operate a computer, schedule a day, remember names and dates, and perform countless other tasks that, once learned, can be repeated automatically without requiring any new learning.

There are some obvious downsides to the reactive mode of thinking. One is that there is no guarantee that what one has learned is actually true and useful. You can and do learn all sorts of things (called beliefs) that were originally learned with insufficient information or perspective. But once learned, the reactive mode of thinking will just automatically assume that the belief is true. It will make its decisions based on that and react accordingly.

Another major downside of this mode of thinking is that when you are in a situation where there is more than one variable that you don't know, your reactive mode of thinking will begin to spin and churn. You will obsess and hash out possible scenarios, never feeling at peace because there are too many unknowns. And where there are unknowns, the reactive mode of thinking will tirelessly try to fill in the holes with faulty assumptions. The result is an energy-draining, frustrating, and stress-creating experience that takes you out of the present moment, into the past or the future, and robs you of peace of mind, effective work in the moment, and even sleep.

Let's use a simple algebra equation as an example. If I gave you the equation $x + 7 = 10$, you would be able to easily solve this and tell me that $x=3$. That was easy because your reactive mode of thinking can solve for one unknown variable. But if I were to give you the equation $x + y = 10$, you would immediately see that this is an unsolvable equation in that there are an infinite number of possible answers $(2 + 8, 1+ 9, -100 + 110)$. You would tell me you couldn't solve the problem until you knew one of the two variables, and you would be right.

But what happens when, instead of a simple algebra equation, you are faced with a situation in your life where there are multiple unknown variables? It could be uncertainty about your job, income, or living situation, or a challenging relationship conflict with your boss, spouse, or child. There may be many different variables that are unknown to you at the moment, and maybe even unknowable for now. But instead of seeing that this is an unsolvable equation until more variables are known, and therefore turning off your reactive processing mode, you instead churn and churn inside. Because it can't solve for multiple unknowns, the reactive mode of thinking will begin to fill in the holes with assumptions that are almost always worst-case scenarios. You impute motive to others' words and actions that you can't possibly know. If your thinking were somehow recorded, it might sound something like this:

"My co-worker took all the credit for that project even though she knew how much I helped. She did that on purpose. She must think I'm an idiot! She must really be out to get me, and what did I do to deserve that? Nothing. In fact, I helped her get where she is today. What a jerk! I'm not going to take that anymore. I'll set her in her place. Or wait, maybe that would make things worse. Maybe I'll just let her have her way for now while I scheme up a way to get back at her and give her what she deserves. But maybe that would show weakness, and I'm always backing away from conflict. What a weakling I am! I wonder why that is? It must have something to do with the way I was raised. My father never really believed in me and never really listened to me. He just wanted me to stay out of the way and not rock the boat. If I ever did, then he would get annoyed and angry with me. It's his fault I'm this way. I hate my father. I hate my co-worker. Actually, I hate myself too. I'm such a loser!"

In the meantime, your son comes in and wants to show you a school assignment that he got a good grade on, and you brush him off with a "Not now. Go show your mom."

The improper use of the reactive mode of thinking when all the variables are not known (churn mode) is the cause of all your stress, worry, anxiety, depression, and sense of hurry and urgency. It is also the cause of your relationship problems, your financial problems, and is even the root source of mental illness and addiction. I know that is a bold statement, but in my experience with myself and with coaching clients, it is always true.

> *Whatever strains with force will soon decay. It is not attuned to the Way.*
> *Not being attuned to the Way, Its end comes all too soon.*
> - LAO TZU

Most of us have been trained to live almost exclusively in the reactive mode of thinking. Our habits, values, beliefs, attitudes, expectations, likes, dislikes, preferences, and even our personality traits are all creations of our reactive mode of thinking.

> *Attention flowing to the past is not energy used; it is energy wasted. The same is true of the future: looking forward to things, worrying about what might happen, fantasizing about dreams coming true is energy drained away. When the mind stays in the present, all this vitality comes back to us.*
> - EKNATH EASWAREN

RECEPTIVE/REFLECTIVE MODE, OR FLOW MODE

The receptive/reflective mode of thinking is sometimes referred to as right-brain thinking. It is a free-flowing mode of thought that is open and receptive to new ideas, new ways of doing things, and new ways of seeing things that the reactive mode of thinking just can't see. It is more like a flowing river than a processing computer. It is the source of original thought, creative intelligence, insight, and wisdom. In flow mode, we have the ability to be open to new ideas and thoughts that we haven't considered before.

Where churn mode is experienced as heavy, busy, or tiring, flow mode is experienced as effortless thinking. It just flows without any real effort on our part. Thoughts and ideas arise easily. In fact, it is an actual, purposeful lack of effort that allows this mode of thinking to arise in our awareness. Our thinking is in the moment, and we experience our awareness as being fully present in the living, breathing moment of now.

> *One who lives in accordance with nature*
> *Does not go against the way of things.*
> *He moves in harmony with the present moment,*
> *Always knowing the truth of just what to do.*
> - LAO TZU

The primary purpose of this mode of thinking is to help us enjoy life, and to operate at peak performance in a fluid, responsive way where we experience ourselves as being an integral part of our environment. We are responsive to whatever is happening or needed in the moment without any need to analyze or solve; we just respond effectively. Professional athletes, inspirational speakers, writers, artists, and teachers often describe a state of being "in the flow" when they experience effortless performance and a feeling of being inspired, as if everything is just flowing through them, not from them. Children at play are frequently in this mode. Their imaginations are flowing and they are living fully in the moment, just experiencing the joy of being alive.

The flow mode of thinking is also the right mode to be in when we're faced with situations where there are many unknown variables. It allows us to stay in a state of peace of mind without the urgency to solve the problem or know the right answer right now. It puts us in a state of trusting that we don't need to know every variable; in fact, knowing all variables would actually be unfulfilling and undesirable. We see that there is so much life to be experienced right here, right now, without anything having to change or be fixed. We miss all of this when we get stuck in churn mode, trying to figure everything out and not being able to rest until we have all the variables solved.

By not wanting, there is calm,
And the world will straighten itself.
When there is silence,
One finds the anchor of the universe within oneself.
- LAO TZU

From this open, receptive state of thinking, we can relax. Relaxing is what allows us to receive new thoughts, insights, and wisdom from the flow of creative intelligence that is always available to us and that we in fact live within, like fish live within the ocean. Whether this flow of creative intelligence comes from the soul or from God or from "the universe" or "source," I don't know; perhaps they're all really the same, and it doesn't really matter. What matters is that it exists and we can tap into it, but only when we're open, quiet and receptive. Only when we're in flow.

You can argue twenty different points of view in intellectual matters,
but with the mysteries of spirit and love, it's best to be bewildered!
In an ocean with no edge, what good are swimming skills?
– RUMI

THE PROPER BALANCE: RECEPTIVE VS. REACTIVE MODE

The receptive mode of thinking is our natural way of thinking. It is our default setting that comes pre-wired. The reactive mode of thinking is also natural to us, but it develops later and is meant to be a tool, used for specific tasks for which it is best suited. It is meant to be turned on when it is the right mode of thinking and then off again when it is not. It is not that one mode is good and the other bad; they are both useful for the right purposes. The difficulty comes when we use reactive thinking in situations far beyond what it was designed for.

We can learn to live in flow mode far more often than we usually do. We can learn to use reactive mode as a tool when necessary, rather than as our dominant and default mode of thinking. The only reason we don't is because we haven't developed enough confidence and trust in the flow and our ability to tap into it effortlessly. Our trust and confidence have too often been placed only in the analytical reactive mode, and that trust is not even well-founded. How many times have you made assumptions and conclusions based on your analytical, reactive thinking that proved to be entirely untrue or grossly exaggerated?

Leave thinking to the one who gave intelligence.
In silence there is eloquence.
Stop weaving, and watch how the pattern improves.
– RUMI

My own sense on the proper balance between the two modes of thinking is that most people spend way too much time stuck in churn mode and not nearly enough time in flow mode. The more stressed-out you are, the more you are stuck in churn mode. It really is that simple. It doesn't matter how much you have on your plate; if you're stressed out, you're stuck in churn mode, whether you're a teenage kid churning over whether your peers like you or the CEO of a Fortune 500 company churning over what your board or investors or peers think of you.

I think the good old 80/20 rule applies here. The proper balance is probably eighty percent of our waking hours in flow mode and only twenty percent in reactive/directive mode (and hopefully very little stuck in churn). The reality for many people is probably the reverse, where eighty-plus percent of their waking hours are stuck in churn mode and twenty percent or less are in flow mode. For many it is more like 90/10 or 95/5, where about the only times they experience flow mode are when engaged in a favorite hobby, exercising, or going on vacation. Even these presumably pleasant activities can be spent stuck in churn mode, as I know I've experienced.

A mind that is fast is sick. A mind that is slow is sound.
A mind that is still is divine.
– Meher Baba

Is there a potential downside to getting stuck in flow mode, like not taking action that needs to be taken? The churn mode of thinking that the personality is prone to get stuck in much of the time actually creates a false fear (illusion) about spending time in flow mode. The fear is that if I (the personality) am not actively trying to fix everything I think needs fixing, I'll just fall into a state of blissful ignorance or avoidance and not accomplish anything, even if I'm no longer stressed out. This line of churn-based reasoning goes on to conclude that stress is actually a good thing, because it's a sign that I'm being productive and have a full plate, and therefore I must be more worthy of self-respect and love. This thought turns out to be just another false conclusion that the personality is skilled at making. The truth is that all great accomplishments and breakthroughs in any field of endeavor are achieved by those people who have learned to turn off the churn mode of thinking when it is not needed, and to trust in the flow of inspiration, guidance, wisdom, and insight that comes from being in the flow mode of thinking.

HOLDING A BASKETBALL UNDERWATER

ANALOGY
Holding A Basketball
Underwater

The wonderful thing to realize about flow mode is that that we don't have to figure out how to turn it on. All we have to figure out is how to turn off our reactive mode when we notice we've gotten stuck in churning. Being in churn mode is the only thing that keeps us from being in flow mode. It's sort of like trying to hold a basketball under water. It takes effort to keep the basketball submerged. But all we have to do is let go, and the natural buoyancy of the basketball allows it to pop up to the surface. It was our effort that kept it down, and our releasing of effort that allowed it to pop up.

When the mind ceases its chatter, the Spirit starts singing.
–Dreaming Bear, Baraka Kanaan

WHAT DOES THIS HAVE TO DO WITH YOGA?

Why did I feel it important to explain our two modes of thinking in a book that is about a five-minutes-a-day, yoga-based, self-care practice? Because the Spiral Up Yoga practice – in addition to all the other things it will do for you – will help you turn off the churn mode of thinking that you're probably stuck in much of the time. It will reconnect you to the natural flow mode in which you want to spend the majority of your time. Doing your five minutes of Spiral Up Yoga every day is like releasing your hold on the submerged basketball and letting it naturally rise to the surface. The more time you can spend in flow mode, the more joyful, creative, and fulfilling your life will be.

Don't worry about getting stuck there. When you're connected to the flow mode of thinking, you'll naturally know how to turn on the reactive/directive mode when it is the right tool for the job at hand. I will make reference to these two modes of thinking throughout the rest of this book, and you'll begin to see all the ways the Spiral Up Yoga practice will help you get unstuck from your overused churning mode and spend more time in your free-flowing receptive mode.

TWO PREREQUISITES TO BEING IN FLOW MODE

I've also found that it is much easier to stay out of churn mode and in flow mode when two things are present:

1. Happiness in the present moment.

2. A positive vision for your future.

These must exist simultaneously. Your happiness cannot be tied to achieving your vision of the future; it must be a present-moment experience, here and now, before you achieve any more of your goals. Since there are two primary criteria, it is sometimes clarifying to construct a simple two-by-two matrix to see what each of the four possible combinations looks like.

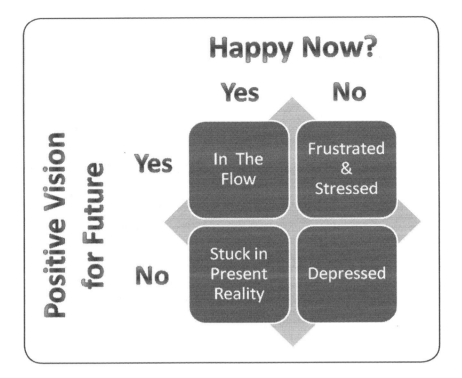

1. **Happy now AND positive vision for your future.** This is the combination that puts you in a state of flow, which not surprisingly, helps you stay in this condition more, creating a virtuous cycle.

2. **Happy now WITHOUT positive vision for your future.** This combination keeps you stuck in your present reality and stifles your growth. One of the ends is blocked up (the outflow end), so it's like you have a dam wall that doesn't allow flow.

3. **Not happy now AND positive vision for your future.** This combination leads to lots of frustration and stress. One of your ends is blocked up (the inflow end), which is like having a dam wall that doesn't allow flow.

4. **Not happy now WITHOUT positive vision for your future.** This dreary combination is a double dam wall blocking both inflow and outflow. This combination quickly leads to depression.

Having Spiral Up Yoga as your foundational self-care practice will create the daily realignment needed to stay happy in the now and have a positive vision of your future. This will allow you to reconnect to your flow mode of thinking on a daily basis. There are other things you can do to get out of churn and into flow, and I work on these with my coaching clients. But without the daily body/mind/soul practice of Spiral Up Yoga, the other things don't have a solid foundation to build on and therefore don't last.

THE ELEVATOR OF CONSCIOUSNESS AND THE HOUSE OF MIRRORS

There is a really great analogy that is very relevant at this point that I'd like to share. I developed this analogy through much of the coaching work that I've done both as a client and as a coach. I have found it to be a very powerful one that once really understood, can be the source of great clarity and peace. I call it the Elevator of Consciousness and The House of Mirrors. It goes like this:

Imagine a tall building with an elevator that can take you up and down between floors. Each level of the building is a house of mirrors. The lower the level of the building, the more distortion there is in the mirrors, and therefore the greater the illusion. The basement floor of the building is completely distorted, and with each floor that you rise, the level of distortion decreases until at the top there is no distortion at all, and you can see clearly, without any illusion.

This analogy describes the human experience on so many levels. Our consciousness can rise and fall, like the elevator. When we are on the lower levels, what we see is very distorted, but we believe it to be "reality," to be "just the way things are." It's not that we are somehow creating distorted thoughts when we're at the lower levels, it's just that those are the quality of thoughts that live at that level, so that's what we see and experience as real. As we rise up through the floors, we experience different thoughts. Again, this is not because we're thinking more positive thoughts, it's simply because these are the quality of thoughts that live at those levels and so that's what we see and experience as real. The higher up we are able to go, the higher the quality of thought that exists there, and the more clearly we see and the more joyful our experience of life is.

When we're at lower levels, we believe the illusions of that level to be "real" and we often make decisions or take actions that seem justified to defend ourselves from what we think we see that is attacking us. These decisions and actions only serve to strengthen the power of the illusion and lengthen the time we spend on the lower floors. They also tend to pull others who are the target of your attacks (that you see as defense) down to the same level of distortion, where each of your actions only serves to further solidify the apparent reality of the illusion.

When we wake up from a dream into waking consciousness, we do not pass from unreality to reality; we pass from a lower level of reality to a higher level. And, the mystics of all religions say, there is a higher level still, compared with which this waking life of ours is as insubstantial as a dream. Yet until we do wake up, nothing sounds more absurd than the assertion that we are dreaming, and nothing seems more solid than this world of the senses. Why should this be so? If original goodness is our real nature, why are we unable to see it? The answer is simple: because we see life not as it is but as we are. We see "through a glass darkly," through the distorting lenses of the mind – all the layers of feeling, habit, instinct, and memory that cover the pure core of goodness deep within.
— Eknath Easwaren

WE ALL GET TO EXPERIENCE THE LOWER LEVELS

I don't know of anyone who doesn't spend some time on the lower levels. It seems to be part of the design of the human experience and evolutionary process that we all get to experience the lower levels. Neither do I think the purpose is to try to avoid them, but rather to learn to see them for what they are – highly distorted and not at all real. When you do happen to be on a lower level (for whatever reason), the best policy is to not believe anything you see and not take any actions, no matter how justified they seem. The less action we take on the lower levels, the quicker our elevator will take us up to higher levels. The more we buy into the reality of the lower levels, the longer we will get stuck there.

HOW TO KNOW YOUR CURRENT LEVEL

ANALOGY
Emotions as Truth Feedback

How do you know what level you're on? As it turns out there are no buttons to push or signs to let you know what floor you're on. The best answer I have discovered is to pay attention to how you feel. Thoughts are very tricky things and you're not always aware of what thoughts you're actually experiencing at any given moment. But you are always aware of how you're feeling. This is part of the kindness of the design. Our emotions give us instantaneous feedback as to the quality of the thoughts we are believing. So while our minds, or more accurately our personalities, can be easily deceived by illusions, our emotions, which are part of the built-in intelligence of the body, can be our guide. It's pretty simple, really; the lousier you feel, the greater the illusion you are believing and therefore the lower the floor you are currently on. The lousier you feel, the less you should trust your perceptions and your reactions, no matter how justified they appear to be.

The best thing you can do at this level is to release your grip on it. Say to yourself (your personality) something like:

"Even though this appears to be real and demands a strong reaction, I'm feeling lousy, so I know it can't be real. Therefore, I'm going to do nothing. I'm not going to argue or defend myself. I'm not going to shame or blame myself or others. I'm going to just wait it out until I can see more clearly, until I can see from a higher level with less distortion. I'll know I'm

doing that because I'll feel a lot better. Then, and only then, I'll decide if there is really a problem that requires any action on my part. If so, the actions that I can see at that higher level will be much better than any I can currently see at this lower level."

HOW TO GET TO A HIGHER LEVEL

Remember the analogy I used earlier about holding a basketball under water? Because of the ball's natural tendency to rise to the surface, it takes effort and energy to hold it under water. It is your effort that keeps it down and your releasing of control that allows it to rise. This is how the elevator of consciousness works. It is your effort and struggle that keep it stuck in the lower levels and your releasing and allowing, without reacting, that enable the elevator to rise up. Like the basketball, its natural tendency is to rise, not to fall.

DISTINCTION
Certainty vs. Clarity

This is a wonderful thing to realize, because you realize that to get to higher levels you don't have to learn new skills and abilities that you don't already have. It's actually the opposite. All the skills and knowledge your personality has accumulated and clings to with certainty are precisely what keep you on the lower levels. To rise to higher levels, you need to begin questioning all the things of which your personality has become so certain. You need to be humble enough to see that your personality doesn't see, and know that your personality doesn't know, no matter how certain it is and how much evidence it has accumulated to prove its case.

DISTINCTION
Evidence: Proof of Truth vs.
Proof that Beliefs are Magnetic

Evidence is not a sign of truth; it is only a sign that beliefs are magnetic and attract their own evidence. Because all your accumulated evidence was collected while you were hanging out on lower levels, be willing to throw it away as suspect.

THE ELEVATOR HAS A MIND OF ITS OWN

We don't always have control of the elevator. We can't just step in and push a button to go where we want to go. Sometimes we can, but often the elevator seems to have a mind of its own. Part of the human experience is getting to experience all the levels so we can get practice seeing through illusions. It allows us to have compassion for ourselves and others. We know that when we're on lower levels, despite our best intentions, or our previous clarity from moments spent at higher levels, it's really easy to believe the illusions we see because they seem so real. When we can see how that happens to us, we can also see how it is equally true for others, and we don't have to react to them when they are taking actions and saying things based on their distorted view of things from being on a lower level.

When we see this, we see that true forgiveness is seeing that there was never really anything to forgive in the first place. The other person said what they said and did what they did not because they were evil, but because they believed an illusion; they were seeing scary things in the distorted mirrors of a lower level. The same is true for all the stupid things you've said or done, even when you supposedly "knew better." So cut yourself some slack, and do the same for others. We're all together on this amazing experience called being human, and we all get to spend some time on the lower floors.

Of course, the more clearly you can see how this all works, the less often you will find yourself on lower floors; and even when you do find yourself there (by paying attention to your emotions), the quicker you'll be able to release your grip and allow the elevator to take you back up.

MMMM

When you are on the upper levels of the elevator, there is an experience that is common to all who spend time there. There is a sense of bewilderment and magic and timelessness of the present moment. I have come to call this "MMMM" moments, which stands for "Magic and Mystery of this Magnificent Moment."

These moments can happen at any time and any place. They are what it feels like when we penetrate the veil of illusions, even for just a moment or two. The experience is beyond words, and about all I can utter is "MMMM." It may be holding my young child in my arms and gazing into her light-filled eyes and really perceiving what a miracle she is, and I am, and how priceless this exact moment is and how blessed I am to be experiencing it. It may be really appreciating the beauty of a sunrise or sunset or the nature around you. It may be just perceiving what a miracle each moment really is. MMMM moments can happen spontaneously, but we can also create them. In truth, MMMM moments are every single moment – it's just a matter of how aware of them we are from moment to moment. I personally make it a daily practice of mine to become aware of several MMMMs each day. If I'm going to bed and haven't noticed one, I can, in that moment, notice the one I'm experiencing right then.

I invite you to make this a daily practice to complement your daily Spiral Up Yoga practice. Make each moment of practicing Spiral Up Yoga, MMMM moments. I teach my coaching clients this principle and have coined a phrase I like to use: "An MMMM or two a day keeps the illusions away."

O wondrous creatures,
By what strange miracle
Do you so often
Not smile?
– Hafiz

PART 3
The Yoga Foundation

⑨
ORIGINS OF YOGA AND THE PERENNIAL PHILOSOPHY

The earliest known references to yoga in Hindu tradition are the Vedas, an oral tradition that Hindu tradition holds as being at least ten thousand years old. Many of the principles of yoga show up in other ancient Hindu texts, including the Ramayana, believed to be about seven thousand years old, the Mahabharata, believed to be about five thousand years old, and the Upanishads, which are about three thousand years old. The most complete, detailed, organized, and written presentation of yoga as a spiritual, mental, and physical practice is found in the Yoga Sutras, written by Maharishi Pantanjali some two thousand five hundred years ago. But the true origins of yoga are really unknown and shrouded in antiquity.

Many believe that the philosophies and practices of yoga were originally revealed to humans by the gods and therefore predate all recorded history. Indeed, the principles that yoga is built on can be found in many other ages and civilizations, including ancient Egyptian, Chaldean, and Asian traditions. The ancient Korean text called the Chun Bu Kyung (the Heavenly Code), which according to Korean tradition dates back ten thousand years, contains very similar principles and teachings, and is believed to have been revealed directly from God. The Asian-based martial arts are ancient practices designed to help the practitioners to find union with the divine within and around them, but it is only possible to realize such unity through the body – not as an intellectual concept or spiritual principle.

Many people assume that the history of humanity is a continual evolution from ape man to modern civilized man. The reality of history is quite different. It is more a series of rather sudden emergences of highly civilized cultures with written language, advanced art and technology, sophisticated government, and extremely advanced building construction knowledge (like the Chaldeans, the Egyptians, the Mayans, the Chinese dynasties, the Aryans, and the Indus) that cannot be explained by gradual evolution. These highly advanced civilizations eventually devolve over the course of many centuries, reverting to lower levels of survival existence, until eventually there is another spike in civilization as a result of timeless principles being revealed or rediscovered by a new people.

Aldous Huxley has called these principles, which are the basis of all mystical traditions and their eventual religious practices, the "perennial philosophy." According to Huxley, the perennial philosophy consists of three principles:

1.   There is an infinite, changeless reality beneath the world of change.

2. This same reality lies at the core of every human being, beneath the level of personality.

3. The purpose of life is to discover this reality experientially; that is, to realize God while here on earth in this body.

Yoga as a lifestyle, a philosophy, and a physical practice is really a personal experiment in realizing for oneself this supreme reality.

You cannot know it, but you can be it, at ease in your own life.
Discovering how things have always been brings one into harmony with the Way.
- LAO TZU

My own definition of yoga is this:

Anything that brings about a realignment and greater union of body, mind and soul and reconnects us to our divine source is yoga.

So you can see that yoga is much more than just a form of physical exercise to increase flexibility. My own definition of yoga is this: anything that brings about a realignment and greater union of body, mind, and soul and reconnects us to our divine source is yoga.

The word "yoga" comes from Sanskrit and has the meaning of unity. It is generally considered to mean a unifying of body, mind, and soul with the greater divine reality. As this happens, we come to see – not just intellectually, but experientially – that we are all divine beings having a human experience. The earliest use of the word "yoga" is from the ancient Rig Veda, which speaks of "yoking (or unifying) the mind to the highest truth."

Over the course of the thousands of years of yoga tradition, yoga has taken many different forms. Today there are many different styles practiced throughout the world – each with its own particular emphasis, but all pointing toward the same perennial philosophy.

A great scholar hears of the Tao and begins diligent practice.
A middling scholar hears of the Tao and retains some and loses some.
An inferior scholar hears of the Tao and roars with ridicule.
Without that laugh, it would not be the Tao.
- LAO TZU

10
WHAT PRACTICING YOGA WILL DO FOR YOU

The benefits of practicing yoga on a regular basis are comprehensive, positively impacting your body, mind, and soul. Modern medical research and testing of yoga practitioners show a host of verifiable benefits to one's health. Many medical practitioners are beginning to take notice and recommending that patients look into practicing yoga to benefit their health on many levels. Yoga is becoming very popular in Western civilization today, with thousands of yoga studios spread throughout the world, both in large cities and in small towns. It's become popular with celebrities; many of them credit yoga with helping them stay in shape physically, mentally, and spiritually. But is it just a fad? If it is, it's a ten-thousand-year-old fad. The fact that yoga has been around in various forms, arguably since the dawn of humanity, is evidence that it is highly beneficial to the human experience. It is only in recent years that it has become more accessible and accepted. Of course, the best way for you to know what the benefits are is to practice it yourself. Intellectually understanding the benefits won't actually benefit you. Experimenting with it and experiencing the benefits in your own life is what will actually sell you on maintaining it as a practice.

Here are just a few of the benefits you can expect from practicing yoga:

BODY

- **Release of Stress and Tension in the Body.** Stress in the mind creates stress in the body, which shows up as tension and constriction. For most of us, tension builds up in the body on a daily basis and, if not released often, can cause chronic dis-ease (disease) in the body. This one benefit alone will have many ripple effects on your health and well-being.

- **Energizing and Relaxing the Body.** It sounds paradoxical, but that is my experience: feeling simultaneously relaxed and energized. It's actually not paradoxical because it is tension held in the body (and created by our thinking) that constricts the natural flow of energy throughout the body.

- **Increased Flexibility.** Most people become less flexible over time. Babies are super flexible, but by the time we're teenagers, we've often lost a lot of our innate flexibility, and by the time we're in our thirties and forties and beyond, it just seems to get worse. But it doesn't have to be this way. Inflexibility is just another result of the buildup of tension in the body, and the consistent practice of yoga, even in very small doses, will restore natural flexibility over time. Flexibility is not just about being able to bend over and touch your toes without bending your knees; it's about feeling free and fluid within your body instead of trapped within it.

- **Pain Relief.** Pain relief is another side effect of the releasing of tension from the body. Pain is often caused by tense muscles, ligaments, and joints which, when relaxed and energized, loosen up. The pain then goes away. Pain is always trying to tell you that something needs attention, and that usually means you need to relax and release tension.

- **Deeper, More Natural Breathing.** A big part of a yoga practice is the breath. If you watch a baby breathe, you'll see that it breathes naturally from the lower belly in slow, deep breaths. As we age, what tends to happen is our breathing gets higher and shallower. Often, people who are dying are breathing rapidly and shallowly and way up in the throat. Yoga practice can help you reverse this trend and return your breathing to more natural, deep-bellied, slow breathing. The breath is also the primary mode of taking in vital energy from our environment – it is not just air we breathe, but energy. Deliberate breath control is one of the core practices of yoga. Of all the vital functions of the body that are controlled by our autonomous systems, breathing is the one thing we can easily take conscious control of. In essence, the breath is the one function that bridges our conscious and subconscious brain functions. Conscious control of the breath can be used in a number of ways, depending upon the desired effect. It can be used to energize and stimulate or to calm and relax. As part of the Spiral Up Yoga system, you'll learn various conscious breath control methods that you can do anytime, anywhere.

- **Greater Strength.** Many of the yoga positions help you develop greater strength, both in your core (abdominals and torso) and in your periphery (arms, legs, and neck). This isn't like lifting weights; you'll never need to worry about getting bulky muscles. But if you want that, you can lift weights, too.

- **Improved Posture and Balance.** The physical yoga positions are designed to help us maintain correct alignment and posture. This is another thing that seems to decline with age, but doesn't need to. Regular practice, even in small doses, will help realign your skeletal structure, which has often gotten out of alignment due to tension in the muscles and ligaments. Balance is another thing that often deteriorates with age. Many people lose their balance easily if they stand on one foot while closing their eyes. Yoga will help to restore you to a more grounded, balanced state.

- **Weight Management.** Yoga helps to release the buildup of cortisol in the body. Cortisol is the stress hormone that triggers fat production as a means of protecting the body from perceived threats. Lower levels of cortisol aid the body in releasing excess weight. Of course there are many factors that impact one's weight, and I am not making any promises of weight loss. But anything that can contribute to less stress, tension, and cortisol in your body is an important step in the right direction. Additionally, I have found that practicing yoga tends to curb my appetite for sweets. I'm giving my body a natural energy boost, so it doesn't tend to crave a sugar-induced one

- **Cardiovascular Conditioning.** Yoga will help you lower your resting heart rate and improve your oxygen intake. It will also help you relax your vascular system, restoring better flow of blood and energy.

- **Lymphatic Circulation and Detoxing.** Your lymph fluid is your body's garbage-disposal service at the cellular level. Lymph fluid and lymph nodes that store lymph don't have their own pump to circulate them (like blood, which has the heart). Lymph is circulated through moving the body, and the various yoga positions help you do that in a way that helps your lymph system to circulate more and detox more.

- **Restoring Proper Energy Flow.** I'll get into more detail on this in the chapter on your energy body, but briefly stated, there is a proper directional flow of energy though the body. This can easily get reversed, like turning counter-clockwise instead of clockwise. This results in many negative side effects until the energy flow is restored to the proper direction.

- **Improved Digestion.** Yoga will also help with your body's digestion and elimination functions. First of all, yoga restores the proper energy flow (mentioned briefly above). This creates the right temperatures in the belly for better digestion. Also, the breath work and movements stimulate the intestines and help them to move waste materials through the system better.

MIND

- **Mental Stress Relief.** Stress originates in our thinking. It begins with an unquestioned belief that things should be other than they are, and therefore I must do something about it to make them the way I think they should be. There are actually lots of different beliefs we tend to adopt early in our lives. When we stop questioning those beliefs, it causes us to create stress for the rest of our lives (until we learn to see things differently, which is a big part of the personal and business coaching that I do). A regular practice of yoga can help create a greater flexibility of mind, not just of body. A big part of the Spiral Up Yoga system is what I refer to as belief upgrading.

- **Greater Clarity, Insight, and Creativity.** Yoga will help you to relax the overactive analytical mind that is the source of all your stress. Yes, the source of all your stress. It is never anything outside of your thinking that is the source of your stress. You don't have to accept this statement. Many will find it too hard to accept because they see the sources of stress as being "out there" in the world – things that happen to them. When you relax your overactive analytical mind, which practicing yoga does for you, you automatically begin to access the intuitive, flow mind that will deliver to you the insights, wisdom, and creativity that is always available to you but cannot be accessed when your analytical mind is churning.

- **Greater Ability to Focus in the Present Moment.** Practicing yoga really forces you to bring your attention from wherever it has been roaming in the past or future and bring it right back into your body in the present moment. The conscious focus on breath, or on holding a position in the body, or on upgrading a belief, or on generating a specific thought that creates a specific emotional response, or toning a sound with your voice, or deeply inhaling a specific aromatherapy oil – all of these activities (which are all part of the Spiral Up Yoga system) help you to be fully present in the moment. This is an innate ability you have, but have likely neglected and need to take back. This ability will help you to live more joyfully in every present moment without the belief that you need to change anything in order to experience enjoyment.

- **Elevated Mood and State of Mind.** One of the most immediate things I notice after doing yoga for a few minutes is that my mood lifts and I go up a notch or two (or more) in my state of mind. It doesn't mean that I never get in a low mood, but when I do, I'm more aware of the fact that it will pass, and the less I try to "fix" it with my analytical thinking, the sooner it will pass. I'm able to see moods more like weather. Sometimes it's sunny and sometimes it's cloudy, and it's all good; it's all part of the beauty of weather. My occasional low moods help me better appreciate the majority of the time, when my mood is elevated. My elevated moods help me have more compassion for myself (and others) when low moods happen (as they inevitably will).

SOUL

- **Greater Connection with Your Soul.** It isn't important to go into too much depth about what the soul really is. Let's just say it's the part of you that existed before your body was formed and will continue to exist after your body is unformed. It is your divine core; the essence of who you really are; the inhabiter of your body. It is the silent partner behind the personality you have come to think of as yourself. It has a sense of purpose and mission; it understands why it's here and what it's here to experience and contribute. I'm not sure that yoga really improves the soul like it improves the body and mind. Rather, I see it as helping create greater unity and alignment of the body and mind to the soul, so that we can feel its presence more and experience more of its natural qualities of love and compassion to self and to others. When we are in this more aligned state, we feel an innate sense of worth and purpose and connection with all others and with all creation. We feel more at one with life and all that is.

- **Deeper Connection with Others.** A natural result of being more connected with your soul is that you also see that everyone you interact with is also a soul (often obscured by an insecure personality) just like you are. Judgments of others fall away and you see the divine in everyone, even if they can't see it yet themselves. You naturally listen to others on a deeper level, hearing what they are really trying to say.

- **Inner Peace.** Yes, yoga will bring you inner peace. It's not so much that it creates it; rather, it allows you to become more aware of it as part of the innate nature of your soul. The peace that you'll feel as part of practicing yoga is not just a greater peace of mind, but also a peace in the body and a peace in the soul. It's the natural result of greater unity between body, mind, and soul, and greater alignment with the divine within you and around you. It is experiencing more fully the sweetness of just being alive and embodied and aware, and aware that you are aware. I often experience it as something like, "Holy cow – I'm alive! I'm here now, in this body, experiencing the breath and energy flow through me and my heart beating and seeing what I'm seeing and hearing what I'm hearing and smelling what I'm smelling and touching what I'm touching, and even having the challenges that I'm having right now so they can make me stronger... Holy cow! This whole human experience is amazing. And I don't have to do anything to earn it – it's just given to me. Now, what was I worried about?"

I don't know of any other form of exercise that can do all of this for me. Nor am I aware of any other spiritual practices that can have such a profoundly positive effect on my body. That's not to say all other forms of exercise or spiritual practice are inferior; it's just that I wouldn't want to let them crowd out my yoga practice. And with Spiral Up Yoga, I don't have to. I can do my yoga practice in five minutes a day and still do other forms of exercise or spiritual practices that I enjoy. The yoga practice is my foundation, and everything else is a nice addition. I know I'm claiming a lot here, but I'm doing it out of my own direct experience over years of practicing. And I'm not asking you to take my word for it; I'm asking you to experiment with it yourself and see what you experience.

A person whose mind is free from negative thinking spreads a life-giving influence in much the same way that a tree gives oxygen. Although a selfless man or woman may seem to go through the day doing nothing extraordinary, without them nothing would revitalize the atmosphere in which we think. By being vigilant, and not encouraging negative thoughts, all of us can offer this vital service – which benefits everybody, including ourselves.

- Eknath Easwaren

But even if the benefits are wonderful, if the practice of yoga requires too much time or is too complex to remember and keep track of, you are likely to never try it, or to try it for a while but not sustain it as a lifelong practice. This is why I felt compelled to create a practice I knew I could sustain for my whole life. Because I knew that five minutes a day over five plus decades (God willing) would be more transformational than two hours twice a week, on and off for a few months, which was my actual experience before creating Spiral Up Yoga.

YOUR THREE BODIES: A BRIEF OWNER'S GUIDE

To better understand what is actually happening when you are practicing Spiral Up Yoga, it's useful to have a basic understanding of your three bodies. Yes, you have three bodies.

Physical Body: That's the one you're mostly aware of and think of as your body.

Energy Body: The energetic body is a larger body of energy that interpenetrates your physical body but also extends beyond it. It plays the intermediary role between your physical body and your spiritual body.

Spirit Body: Some traditions refer to the spiritual body as the causal body. Your spirit body interpenetrates your energy and physical bodies but also extends beyond them. The spirit body is the seat of awareness and consciousness and is the enlivening cause of what we call life.

THREE BODIES NESTING DOLL

ANALOGY
Three Bodies Nesting Doll

You might think of your three bodies like a nesting doll, where one doll fits inside the next larger one. Many people think of their spirits as dwelling within their bodies, but have you ever considered it might be the other way around: that your body dwells within your spirit?

Once again, I'm not asking you to take my word for any of this. It's not even important that you really understand the details of how it all fits together. Instead, just take this as a personal experiment to explore for yourself.

PHYSICAL BODY

Of the three bodies, the physical body is well understood at its basic mechanical level. Yet even with all the amazing miracles of modern-day medicine and technology, our collective understanding of the physical body is minute compared to what is not yet understood. What is clear to me (even though you'd never find it in modern medical establishment texts) is that the physical body is at the end of the chain of cause and effect. It is the physical reflection of the subtler energy body and spirit body. As such, it seems clear to me that limiting your perception of cause and effect to only the physical body as a self-contained and separate unit is extremely limiting. This is why the placebo effect is such an inconvenient truth to the medical establishment. They can't argue its huge impact on the physical body, but they can't explain it, either, other than a tacit acknowledgment that the mind does seem to be able to trick the body.

ENERGY BODY

The energy body is understood even less than the physical body, but the ancient yoga traditions of India and their similar counterparts in other ancient cultures all teach of an energy body that can actually be sensed by our physical body's senses. There have always been some people who have either been born with or developed heightened sensory perceptions that can see and feel energy bodies (sometimes called auras). Actually we can all perceive energetic fields around others, even if we're not consciously aware of it. For example, we are attracted to people with really loving, expansive energy bodies. Conversely, our internal warning bells go off when someone approaches us who is in a dark place energetically and is feeling compelled to do physical harm. We've all experienced a drain on our energy when we've been around others who are depressed or despondent, and we've all experienced a boost of our energy when we've been around someone who is really upbeat and enthusiastic. There was no pill ingested or shot injected, but we most definitely felt the effect.

In fact, whether you're consciously aware of it or not, your energy body is interacting with, impacting, and being impacted by the energy bodies of everyone and everything you interact with. It is also responding to the quality of your thinking all the time. This is why when you believe a worrisome or anxious thought, you can feel your energy constrict. Your physical body follows suit, hunching your neck and shoulders as if to protect yourself from a hidden blow to the back. Likewise, when you believe a thought that is exciting and fun to you, you can feel your energy expand. You may find yourself automatically pumping your fist in the air and doing a little happy dance while you shout "Yes!"

Modern-day technology is just recently beginning to "see" the energy body. Kirlian photography is able to capture energy-field images – not just around human bodies, but around plants, animals, and even minerals. In all cases, the energy body both interpenetrates and extends beyond the physical body. Want to see what it looks like? Just do an image search on the Internet for "Kirlian photography" and see what comes up.

I'm going to go into more detail on the energy body in the next chapter, because having a deeper understanding of the energy body will make your practice of Spiral Up Yoga much more fascinating and enjoyable. The whole structure of the Spiral Up Yoga system is based on chakras, which are an important part of the energy body.

SPIRIT BODY

Even less is understood about the spirit body, but once again, all the ancient traditions speak of a spirit body or soul that is eternal and timeless. In its presence there is life and an organizing intelligence of the matter and energy that make up the physical body and energy body. Without its presence there is death and disintegration in the physical and energy bodies, and the matter that was organized into the physical body begins to disintegrate into basic matter that can then be recycled and used by spirit to create other physical bodies.

Most religions teach of the existence of a spirit or soul that is eternal. But once again, you don't have to take my word for it, or even the word of all the world's religions. You can experience your spirit body directly and know that it is. I guarantee you that you've already experienced this many times, but you may not be consciously aware of it now. Yoga helps you to become more aware of the presence and influence of your spirit body, or soul, that is always there with you. In fact, your spirit body is who you truly are beneath your personality and your physical body, which are both just temporary creations of your spirit body.

Modern biomedical scientists can manipulate DNA and synthesize tissues, but by themselves the tissues are inert and just sit there in a petri dish, lifeless. Scientists still need to insert living organic tissue to enliven the engineered tissues. There is a spark of life they cannot engineer – a spiritual, invisible life force that must be introduced before the organic material becomes living matter.

Yoga recognizes all three bodies and also recognizes the chain of causality starting with spirit, which is then translated into energy, which is then translated into the physical. The proper practice of yoga brings our awareness to all three bodies living together in a divine union we call being human.

When you look for it, there is nothing to see.
When you listen for it, there is nothing to hear.
When you use it, it cannot be exhausted.
-Lao Tzu

THE "I AM" EXPERIMENT

EXPERIMENT
The "I Am" Experiment

I love this experiment to help me get a real sense of my own "I-am-ness." Take a few minutes now and try this yourself. Get to a place where you can be alone and not interrupted for a few minutes. Look around wherever you are and begin a self-inquiry process as follows:

Q: What are you experiencing right now in this moment? Notice everything you notice.

Q: Who is aware that I am experiencing what I am experiencing? I am.

Now go back to five minutes ago.

Q: What was I experiencing five minutes ago?

The content of my thoughts was different. I may have been in a different place. Billions of my cells have replaced themselves since then, but I am that same awareness that was aware five minutes ago.

Now go back five hours ago.

Q: What was I experiencing five hours ago?

There has been even greater change in the last five hours. Yet one thing has not changed. I am still the one who was aware of whatever I was experiencing five hours ago.

Now five years ago.

Q: What has changed? What has stayed the same?

Now fifty years ago (even if has not been fifty years since your physical birth).

Q: What has changed? What has stayed the same? Where you still aware of whatever you may have been experiencing fifty years ago, whether in this body and personality or before?

Now try five hours from now.

Five years from now.

Fifty years from now.

Five hundred years from now.

Everything changes; the content of your thoughts, the physical surroundings you find yourself in, the people you find yourself with, the things you find yourself doing, even the state of being embodied in this physical body or not. But one thing still remains constant and unchanging; your I-am-ness, your awareness of experiencing whatever you are experiencing. This is the essential you, the eternal you that has always been and always will be. Really try to feel the presence of your eternal nature. Now ask yourself these questions:

Q: How does your perspective on your problems change?

Q: Where do your feelings of stress and anxiety come from?

Q: What are you scared of?

Q: What do you lack?

Q: What is stopping you?

This is a great experiment to conduct whenever you start to lose perspective of who you really are, which is always the case when you're feeling stressed, inadequate or anxious. I recommend this as one of the activities for the Seventh Chakra day (Sundays). Spend a few minutes each Sunday just doing this experiment. It won't take more than a few minutes once you get used to doing it, and it will serve to strengthen your connection to your own soul.

Just sit there right now
Don't do a thing
Just rest.
For your separation from God
From love,
Is the hardest work
In this world.
– Hafiz

My mention of Moses may block the message, if you think I refer to something in the past.
The light of Moses is here and now, inside you. Pharaoh as well.
– Rumi

YOUR ENERGY BODY: A BRIEF OWNER'S GUIDE

Understanding more about your energy body will make your practice of yoga more meaningful. It will also allow you to become aware of more of what is really happening on a moment-by-moment basis with your health, your moods, your energy levels, and your interactions with other people (and even with other forms of life like animals and plants).

Work in the invisible world at least as hard as you do in the visible.
– RUMI

A QUICK EXPERIMENT: FEELING YOUR ENERGY BODY

Before going into more detail about your energy body, I'd like you to first conduct a little experiment to see if you can actually feel your energy body. It's a simple exercise and should only take a minute or two.

The palms of the hands are the most sensitive receptors for feeling the energy body. This is why, if you've ever watched or experienced anyone conducting energy work, you'll see they use their open palms to feel the energy body as well as to transmit energy to the other person. Place the palms of your hands facing each other a few inches apart. Close your eyes so that you can focus your awareness on your sense of touch. Begin consciously breathing slow, deep breaths in your lower belly and consciously relax the muscles in your arms and hands. Try to quiet your analytical mind by assuring it that you only need a minute or so of quiet. Even if you can't quite quiet your analytical mind, remove your attention from the thoughts arising in it and focus your attention and awareness on the space between your palms. Keep your attention on the space between your palms – not in a highly concentrated way, but in a relaxed way. If you become aware of thoughts, don't follow them, just let them come and go without pulling your attention away.

What do you notice? What can you feel in your palms? Most people describe a sensation of tingly energy or a magnetic push or pull sensation. Now begin to slowly expand the space between your palms as you breathe in and contract the space as you breathe out. What do you notice? Did the sensations become a little stronger?

Now, take one palm and place it a few inches above your opposite arm, slowly moving it up and down the arm. Do you feel anything? This is a little harder to feel at first because you're only using one palm receptor instead of two. If you aren't feeling anything through any of this, don't worry – you do have an energy body. It's probably just because your thinking is too loud and still has too much control over your awareness. Practicing yoga will help to loosen the grip your thinking has over your awareness. For many, this is a new concept that awareness and thinking are two very different things.

Now try to enhance the energy in your palms by vigorously rubbing them together until you feel a sensation of heat, and then try the exercise again. This isn't cheating; it's just increasing the energy radiance of your palms so that it becomes easier to sense your energy body. Hopefully you were able to have an experience of actually feeling your energy body. The energy body is much subtler than the physical body, and the spirit body is subtler than the energy body. But both can actually be sensed and experienced by the physical body because the physical body is connected to and interpenetrated by the energy body and spirit body. It's really just a matter of developing a greater sensitivity to subtle energies, which comes as you get better at quieting the chatter of the personality and your ability to do that will be enhanced through your daily practice of Spiral Up Yoga.

ANCIENT KNOWLEDGE OF THE ENERGY BODY

The existence of the energy body and the understanding of its makeup and functioning is actually ancient knowledge that has been available for many thousands of years. It is the basis of Chinese medicine and acupuncture, of martial arts, of Japanese Reiki, and of yoga. The fact that our modern Western medical community is only just recently beginning to acknowledge there might actually be a subtle energy field around the body doesn't mean that the knowledge is new. So while you probably won't find what I'm about to teach you in articles approved by the American Medical Association, you will find plenty of supporting materials from lots of other sources dating back thousands of years.

MAKE UP OF YOUR ENERGY BODY

ANALOGY
Energy Body: City Bus System

Your energy body has three major parts to it: chakras, meridians, and the aura. A useful way to think of these three parts is this: chakras are like central bus stations, and meridians are like the roads that connect the bus stations and branch out to serve the surrounding areas. The aura is like the outside border or envelope within which all the bus stations and roads exist.

PRANA

The energy itself, which flows and circulates through your energy body, is known by different names, like prana (Sanskrit), chi (Chinese) or ki (Korean). Since we're using the Sanskrit word "chakra," I'll stick with the Sanskrit word, "prana." Prana is the subtle energy that flows within our bodies and also throughout the universe. Prana is a receptive form of energy, not an active one. It is intelligent in and of itself, but it is neutral by nature. It must be acted upon by an activating power, and that activating power is the soul, or spirit body.

Therefore the energy body really becomes the medium through which we can experience and realize the spirit body. What this means is that the more sensitized you become to the flow of prana in and around you, the more you will be able to experience your soul, which is eternal life that exists in and of itself. Go back and re-read the last few sentences. What I've just stated is so important that I invite you to really soak it in and reflect on it.

Quantum physicists study the physics of the subatomic. In the last few decades they have been able to see further and further into life at the subatomic level. One of the things they've discovered is that space that was previously believed to be empty is not at all empty, but rather full of a constant and dynamic eruption of energy particles that are intelligent and interconnected. They are still trying to create their own names for what they are discovering, but you and I can just call it what it's been called for thousands of years: prana.

EXPERIMENT: SEEING PRANA

On a clear day with a blue sky, go outside. There can be some light clouds, just so long as there are large patches of blue sky. Stand with your back to the sun and softly focus your gaze about twenty feet in front of you into the blue sky. Keep your focus relaxed – you should not feel any strain on your eye muscles – but bring your full attention to your eyesight and the space you are gazing at. At first you might notice black, floating hair-like or cell-like objects. Don't pay attention to those, as they are actually part of your eyeball. Just keep gazing softly until you begin to see a mass of whitish colored specks that are spinning, popping, and swirling. These are in the air, not an optical illusion within your eye or optic nerve. Is this prana that you are seeing? I believe it is as close as you can see prana with the naked eye. The popping, swirling, spinning characteristics are very similar to what quantum physicists report seeing within empty space at the subatomic level using sophisticated magnification instruments. I only share this little experiment because I find it interesting myself and hope you will too. However, even if you don't see anything like I describe, or if you believe it is just an optical illusion, it isn't really important. Whether prana can be seen or not, it can definitely be felt and practicing Spiral Up Yoga a little bit each day will help you become more sensitive to feeling prana, both within you and around you.

CHAKRAS

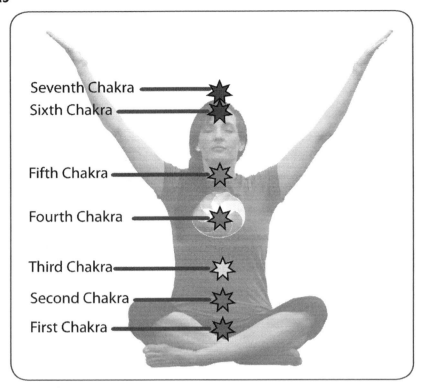

Seventh Chakra
Sixth Chakra
Fifth Chakra
Fourth Chakra
Third Chakra
Second Chakra
First Chakra

There are seven major internal points of intersection for the flow of prana in the energy body. These major intersections or collecting pools are called chakras. There are also four external chakras: one in each palm and in the sole of each foot, but these are secondary. The word "chakra" comes from Sanskrit and means "wheel" or "circle." This is because energy tends to swirl in a circular, spiraling motion as it gathers. Your chakras are spinning pools of energy that vibrate at certain frequencies. They are located at certain places within your energy body, which, because it interpenetrates your physical body, means your chakras are located within your physical body too. A surgeon would never see them if he opened you up, just like he wouldn't see your soul, because they exist at a subtler level than physical matter. Chakras are like rechargeable batteries in the sense that they store energy and then send out the energy through the meridians to service the entire physical body. As such, chakras can wax and wane in their strength and vibrancy. They can even become blocked and backed up, like collecting ponds that get too much debris trapped in the inlets and outlets and begin to stagnate.

Problems in your chakras translate directly into problems in your physical body as well as in your state of mind and moods.

It is not an exaggeration to say that complete health begins and ends with the chakras.

CHAKRAS AS ELECTRICAL SWITCHES TO THE BRAIN

The seven major chakras are also directly linked to different areas of the brain. Using the analogy of turning on a light, the prana is the electricity; the chakras are switches that when turned on will activate different parts of the brain. In a sense, it's like awakening more of the brain. Modern brain researchers believe we only use a small percentage of our brain and much of its potential lies dormant. I believe that as we fully turn on the chakra switches, more of our brains will become awakened and activated.

Your chakras are also intimately involved in your spiritual growth. In the ancient Korean tradition of Shin-Sun-Do (way of the divine), which modern day Dahn yoga is based on, it is taught that in order for the human being to become one with the divine spirituality within, the whole brain must be awakened. This can only happen when all seven chakras are fully activated. This is referred to as "small universe," a state in which all of the chakras are activated, all meridians of the body flow freely, and the mind and body become one. "Great universe" is the state in which cosmic prana and energy-body prana merge into a unified flow, which allows the personal experiential realization of the true self. In the book Healing Chakras by Dahn yoga founder Ilchi Lee, it states:

> "To experience and understand the chakras means that you understand the flow of life, including the meaning of life and death. You might possess the most precious of gems, yet, if you don't know its value, then there is no difference between the gem and an ordinary pebble. One of the primary reasons that people are in constant search for 'meaning' in life is that they don't understand the chakra system within their own bodies. Understanding the True Self, and thereby life's meaning and purpose, lies in an understanding of the chakras. Experiencing the chakras will bring about an overall understanding of life."

Still think yoga is just another form of physical exercise?

MERIDIANS

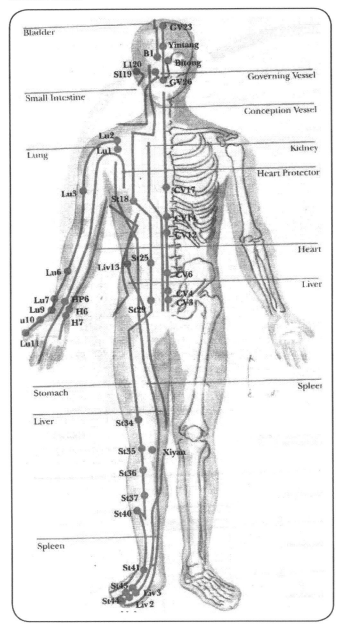

Meridians are the energy paths or channels that extend from the chakras to service the energy body and the physical body. Prana flows through the meridians. Many of the meridians are closer to the outer surface (skin) of the physical body. The ancient Chinese practice of acupuncture works by using needles that penetrate the skin in specific areas, stimulating and unblocking prana flows that may have become restricted. If you've ever tried acupuncture, as I have, it doesn't hurt at all, which means that the meridian system is different from the nervous system. Meridians also run deep within the body and connect with the chakras. Meridians are similar to blood vessels in that there are some that flow in one direction (yang) and others that flow in the opposite direction (yin), much like arteries and veins. The yang meridians are also called sun meridians, and the yin meridians are called earth meridians. There are fourteen major meridians in all.

It's not really important for the purposes of practicing Spiral Up Yoga to have a detailed understanding of all the meridians and their flows and locations. The important thing to know is that by doing the asanas (physical yoga positions), you are stimulating and activating your meridians and your chakras.

Just by spending five minutes a day doing the asanas, by the end of the week you will have done something to strengthen and open the flow for each of your fourteen meridians, seven internal chakras, and four external chakras.

AURA

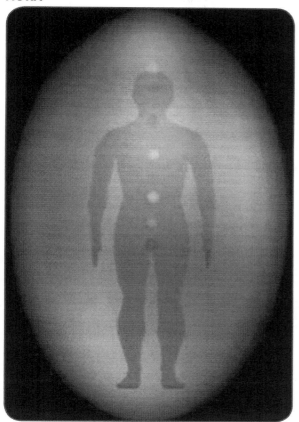

Your aura is like the skin of your energy body. It is generally shaped sort of like an eggshell that surrounds the physical body. It can expand and contract based on the overall health and vibrancy of your energy body, as well as by consciously directing your attention to your aura. The aura is a reflection of the state of health of the chakras, and those who can see auras report that they reflect the various colors emanating from the chakras. Kirlian photography can capture the aura and make it visible to us. Because the state of health of your chakras is constantly changing and your balance of yin and yang energy is constantly in flux, the size, shape, and vibrancy of your aura is always changing. Severely compromised chakras will show up in the aura as brown or black spots, or as holes in the protective shell of the aura.

The size, shape, colors, and brightness of your aura are a reflection of the overall health of your energy body. The size of your aura, in terms of how far it extends beyond your physical body, is a reflection of how much energy you radiate around you. Powerful auras can be sensed by others and can serve to strengthen the auras of other people you come in contact with. Weak auras don't extend very far from the physical body and are a sign of overall low energy and beliefs of low self-esteem or self-worth. The shape of your aura is indicative of how balanced your energy body is. A balanced energy body will have a symmetrical, round shape, while unbalanced energy bodies will have oval or irregular shapes. The brightness of your aura indicates the overall strength of your chakras. The more open and radiating your chakras are, the brighter your aura will be. Dark auras are a sign of chronically stressed chakras.

Even though the aura is constantly changing as a reflection of the constantly changing chakras, the changes are usually incremental, not wildly jumping all over the place. We each have a predominant color in our auras that tends to stay stable over long periods of time, but that too can evolve as we grow. The predominant colors in our auras reflect our personality type or traits. This is really what is at the core of the various personality typing systems and why many of them tend to use colors as the personality categories. Because

I understand that we can and do evolve and transcend limited beliefs and conditioning, and because I know that the practice of yoga is a powerful tool in helping us to do that, I also know that what we think of as a personality type is not nearly as solid or fixed as we sometimes believe it is.

EXPERIMENT: STRENGTHENING YOUR AURA

EXPERIMENT
Strengthening Your Aura

Your aura is primarily a reflection of the health of your chakras, but there are some simple ways you can temporarily increase the strength and vibrancy of your aura. Try this little experiment and see if you notice a difference in how you feel. You can try doing this before entering a room of people, and see if they react differently to you. First you might try not doing it, and seeing how people react, and then leaving and doing it and then re-entering, and seeing if you get a different reaction. People are sub-consciously sensitive to auras. They will likely not know what has happened; they will just respond differently.

Take four slow, deep breaths, imagine you as you do that you are breathing in bright white energy from a ball of white energy sitting above the crown of your head. As you deeply breathe in this white energy, visualize your aura expanding and becoming brighter.

That's it. It's simple. It takes just a few seconds. See what happens.

FIRE DOWN, WATER UP

There is a really useful principle to know about when it comes to determining if your energy body is functioning well or not. This comes from the Dahn yoga tradition and is called fire down, water up. This means that when your energy body is functioning well and energy is flowing smoothly and in the right directions without any significant blockages, you feel relaxed and peaceful, while at the same time alert and energized. Your lower torso, feet and hands will be warm (fire down) and your upper body, especially the neck and head, will be cool (water up). Think of the phrases "fire in the belly" and "a cool head." When in a fire down, water up state, your mouth will be moist, with plenty of saliva; your saliva will taste sweet, and your nasal passages will be open and clear. Your food will digest properly, and your elimination will be regular and pain free. This is the optimal state of health.

But due to stressful thinking, neglect of the energy and physical bodies, and poor eating and drinking habits, this optimal state frequently becomes compromised and the energy flow can become sluggish, blocked, and even reversed. When reversed (water down, fire up) we experience heat and constriction in the neck and head. This leads to a stiff neck and shoulders, headaches, and a dry mouth as the heat literally dries up the saliva in the mouth. Other signs of being in reverse flow include poor digestion, acid reflux, bloating, and irregular and painful elimination.

Our energy body flow state also has a strong influence over our thinking processes. When in proper fire down, water up mode, our analytical/processing minds are relaxed. We naturally revert to flow thinking and we experience peace of mind, gratitude, and natural confidence. When in reverse mode, our analytical/processing minds become overactive and dominate our thinking, blocking out the insight and wisdom that come from being in a relaxed, flow thinking mode. This means that we see fewer options and perceive more threats to our well-being. From this state of mind we tend to make poor decisions and take actions motivated by a sense of urgency that often only make situations worse.

I have a rule of thumb that comes from this understanding I've just taught you. It is this:

Never make an important decision or have an important conversation with a dry mouth.

If I am experiencing a dry mouth, it is mostly likely because I have left my optimal state of energy flow. This means my decision-making ability is temporarily compromised and I don't have access to my wisdom. I am likely to say things to others that will not help and take actions that will be counter-productive and create more problems than they solve.

DAILY ALIGNMENT

The energy balance and flow of the energy body are sensitive and can quite easily get disrupted, blocked, and reversed on a daily basis. Yoga is one of the best ways to address this fact and to restore the energy body to a proper flow. This is why I wanted to create a daily yoga practice that I could sustain. Just practicing yoga once in a while for an hour, while helpful, didn't allow me to restore my energy body to its proper flow on the daily basis that it really needed.

We are shaped by what gains our attention and occupies our thoughts. Today, amidst all of the conditioning to the contrary, we need constant reminders of our higher nature... The media drown us in such a low image of the human being that it is essential to remind ourselves constantly of something higher.
— Eknath Easwaren

HOW I FEEL PRE/POST YOGA SESSION

Pay attention to how you feel after practicing yoga for a clue as to what practicing yoga does for your energy body. With many other forms of physical exercise, I am left with a dry and thirsty mouth. But when I practice yoga, I am left with a moist mouth. See if you experience the same thing.

YOUR SEVEN MAJOR CHAKRAS: WINDOWS TO YOUR SOUL

· ·

The seven chakras are the key to the health of the physical body, the health of the energy body, and even the connection and awareness of the spirit body. In fact, it is impossible to reach a state of enlightened awareness of your true self (your soul) unless the seven major chakras are in good health. So let's explore these chakras. Each one has distinctly different characteristics and impact on our health, our thinking, and even our spiritual development.

The seven major chakras are located deep within the body, generally along the line of the spinal cord. They can be approximated by bringing their locations straight forward to a point on the surface of the physical body.

PHYSICAL BODY IMPACT

Even though I list physical body symptoms that can be attributed to a weak or blocked chakra, I am not advocating that all physical body symptoms and diseases can be cured through chakra work alone. What I am advocating is that chakra work not be ignored in any efforts to heal the physical body. By the time the damage shows up in the physical body, it usually means that the chakra has been weak and compromised for a long time and is probably operating well below fifty percent of optimal health. I am not a doctor, so if you are experiencing physical body symptoms, you should seek medical advice and make your own best decisions. Many doctors are beginning to recommend yoga as a helpful form of self-care for the body. Medical evidence from studies shows irrefutable proof that yoga improves health on so many levels. Most doctors are likely not trained in the energy body and chakras, but if they keep up with medical journals, they will know that yoga is a wonderful way to support the natural healing drive of the physical body. Even if your doctor prescribes medications, nutritional supplements, or surgery, you can safely add chakra work to improve your results. Ultimately, if the chakras are not healthy, the physical body can't and won't be healthy, no matter how much medication or supplementation you ingest or surgery you undergo.

PHYSICAL DISEASES: MAGNET BENEATH THE PAPER

Often, if the underlying energetic cause is not restored to proper balance, chronic diseases that are treated at the physical intervention level alone will recur after a short while in a similar form or a new form. To better see how this works, do a little thought experiment with me. Imagine you have a bunch of metal filings on top of a piece of paper. Underneath the paper is a magnet that is shaped like a square. This invisible magnetic force causes the metal filings to form the visible shape of a square on top of the paper. Let's assume that you want the shape to be a circle, not a square, but you only see what's above the paper. You take a knife and you cut away the edges of the square and try to form a circle. But before long, the metal filings have returned to form a square. If all you ever look at is what you can see with your eyes above the surface of the paper, this will be an endlessly frustrating process. You might come up with a circular shaped barrier to place around the metal filings, but without the barrier in place, the filings will return to the shape of a square. The analogy is hopefully obvious. The metal filings represent the cells of your physical body. The paper represents the barrier between the visible world of matter and the invisible world of energy. The magnet represents the illusionary beliefs we hold about ourselves.

WINDOWS TO YOUR SOUL

The qualities of a person with a strong or weak chakra listed in the upcoming section on each chakra are my own opinions and observations and are by no means comprehensive. The qualities are essentially degrees to which the innate and natural qualities of the soul are allowed to express themselves in your everyday experience of life. I see the strength and openness of a chakra as the size of the window through which the soul can shine in that area. Each of the seven chakras allows different qualities of the soul to shine forth, but the soul is one. It's very much like what happens when pure light is refracted: it is divided into a full-color spectrum that we call the rainbow. The colors of the chakras, not surprisingly, follow the same refraction sequence we see in rainbows: from the lowest visible frequency (red) to the highest (violet), the actual order being red, orange, yellow, green, blue, indigo, and violet.

SUBTRACTING INTERFERENCE

The process of opening and strengthening your chakras is a process of subtraction rather than addition. It is not about adding new knowledge and skills onto a blank slate. It is rather about subtracting and removing any interference and crustiness that has developed over time to weaken our connections with our souls through our chakras.

To remake ourselves, we don't have to bring goodness, love, fearlessness, and the like from without and force them into our hearts somehow. They are already present in us, deep in our consciousness. If we work to remove the impediments that have built up over many years of conditioning, to dislodge the old resentments and fears and selfish desires, our life will become like a fountain of living waters, as it was meant to be.
An old fountain may be clogged so that not much water can get through. But with a lot of cleaning, you can get the water to start playing again. Then grass and flowers will grow around it, and birds will come there to have their bath. Just so, love can flow from us as from a living fountain, and those we live and work with will come to us to be refreshed.
- EKNATH EASWAREN

All of the tools I share with you as part of the Spiral Up Yoga system are designed to help you subtract interference that has built up, thus opening up your connection to your soul and allowing a greater expression of the amazing qualities of your soul. Your chakras are brightly colored lights within you that connect you to your soul, but these lights get covered in silt and dirt and debris, and the light becomes dimmer and the connection to the soul becomes cloudy and weak. Spiral Up Yoga is designed to help you scrape away a little bit of the dirt from one chakra each day. At the end of the week, you'll have done some internal cleaning of all seven lights. Then you repeat that process each week, eventually removing all the accumulated dust and dirt so the lights shine brightly and powerfully, like they were meant to. Of course, just like dust accumulates on a daily basis, you pick up interference or "chakra dust" on a daily basis, but the Spiral Up Yoga practice is like keeping your chakras dusted and clean on a daily basis.

> *Learning consists of daily accumulating.*
> *The practice of the Tao consists of daily diminishing;*
> *Decreasing and decreasing, until doing nothing.*
> *When nothing is done, nothing is left undone.*
> *True mastery can be gained*
> *By letting things go their own way.*
> *It cannot be gained by interfering.*
> - LAO TZU

INNATE ENLIGHTENMENT

The process of removing the dust and crustiness from your chakras is a process that leads to what I call innate enlightenment. What I mean by innate enlightenment is that your enlightenment is already innate within you; it just needs to be uncovered and allowed to shine forth. Enlightenment doesn't come, as many imagine, from seeking out knowledge that you don't have. It doesn't come from journeying to far lands or sitting at the feet of enlightened gurus, or reading libraries of books on enlightenment. I'm not suggesting that these external seeking ways can't contribute to one's own enlightenment process, but they are not sufficient of themselves. The best they can do is to help the seeker to see that true seeking is always within, not without.

> *There is about wisdom a nobility and magnificence in the fact that she doesn't just fall to a person's lot, that each man owes her to his own efforts, that one doesn't go to anyone other than oneself to find her.*
> - SENECA

The way of illumination seems dark,
Going forward seems like retreat,
The easy way seems hard,
True power seems weak,
True purity seems tarnished,
True clarity seems obscure,
The greatest art seems unsophisticated,
The greatest love seems indifferent,
The greatest wisdom seems childish.
- LAO TZU

INTERNAL DIMMER SWITCH

ANALOGY Internal Dimmer Switch

Enlightenment is literally allowing the light within you to shine forth. Enlightenment cannot be learned intellectually, and it cannot be given from one person to another. Enlightenment is really just what happens as you begin to see more from the eyes of your soul and allow the innate qualities of your soul to shine forth. When you subtract enough interference to your own innate enlightenment, you become more enlightened. Enlightenment is not something that you either have or not. It is a continuum, like an infinite dimmer switch within you. The more interference you remove, the more your soul can shine forth, and the more enlightened you are. But just like a dimmer switch can turn up and down, if you allow the dust to accumulate and dim your light within, you become less enlightened.

To know humanity, understand earth.
To know earth, understand heaven.
To know heaven, understand the Way
To know the Way, understand the great within yourself.
- LAO TZU

YOUR PERSONAL FALL FROM GRACE AND YOUR REBIRTH

Little babies are born with bright, open chakra windows. Without speaking, they can instantly bypass our carefully guarded personalities, open our hearts, and connect directly to our souls. This is something that is universally observable. You've probably experienced it yourself as you've held a baby. For sure if it were your own, but even if it were not your own child, you've likely experienced this many times. I remember when our first-born son, Kyle, was about six months old, we travelled to Hong Kong to visit my parents who were living there at the time. Everywhere we went with him, we were stopped by people passing by on the crowded streets. Their eyes would light up and they would pinch his chubby cheeks and speak in words we couldn't understand, but we knew what they meant. It was just the natural response of a soul in an adult body being directly touched by another soul in a brand new baby body.

It might be hard to believe, but you too had that power of instant soul-to-soul connecting when you were a little baby. What happened? I see it like this: we are each born into our own Garden of Eden state where our spirit bodies, energy bodies, and physical bodies are aligned and unified with bright, open, strong chakras holding them all together. Then we each go through our own personal fall from grace as we become socialized and conditioned by our world and lend our belief to the illusions that those around us seem to believe. We each partake of the fruit of knowledge, which means we internalize the beliefs of our society about what is good and bad. We become certain that things are the way they appear to us.

We can live in this fallen state for the rest of our earthly lives, but we don't have to. We can little by little begin uncovering our chakras from all the illusions that have covered them up. As we begin to remove the illusions and expose the light that has always been shining brightly beneath it, we experience a new awakening, a new birth. We experience our souls more fully. The soul has always been there, whispering and guiding, but never forcing; patiently awaiting our voluntary choice to begin scraping away at all the accumulated crustiness that has kept us in a state of relative disconnection from our souls.

The soul can and does break through on rare occasions, and we can have moments of significant spiritual awakening or profound peace and tranquility. But those moments, as wonderful as they are, usually don't have a lasting effect on our daily experience of life. The crustiness of our limiting beliefs sets back in, and if we don't have an effective daily practice (like Spiral Up Yoga) to reverse the accumulation of crustiness, it doesn't take long before we're back to where we were before the pinnacle moment, and maybe even lower.

The accumulation of crustiness happens on a daily basis, so we must have a daily practice to offset and counteract it. You now have a very powerful one in Spiral Up Yoga!

I do believe the soul-smothering effect of childhood can be minimized, but probably not avoided, by higher-consciousness parenting. This is one of the things I really love to work on with my coaching clients that are parents, no matter how old their children are, because it is never too late to be a more conscious parent.

Right now in the darkness there is a voice asking you a question:
Do you remember?
If the answer is yes,
When you open your soul to speak, Light will be born.
If the answer is no,
Then the question just keeps on repeating,
For the Lover is always waiting,
With infinite patience at your Heart's doorstep,
Searching intently in your eyes for a sign
Of even the vaguest recognition of the happiness you once shared,
Before you hit your head on the overhand of ego's awning
And caught amnesia of all you once were.
- DREAMING BEAR, BARAKA KANAAN

INTERCONNECTED SPECTRUMS

Different qualities of your soul are either blocked or allowed to shine forth through different chakras. As you read through the following chapter that discusses details of each of your seven chakras, keep in mind that when I share the qualities of someone with a strong or weak chakra, this is to give you an understanding of two ends of a spectrum. Begin to notice where on the spectrum you might currently be for each of your chakras. Please know that no matter where you are currently, you have within you the innate potential to open and strengthen your chakras. As you do, the qualities associated with having that chakra be strong will automatically become part of your experience. Also, the qualities of the seven chakras, while they are organized by chakra, are quite interconnected. As you open and strengthen your connection with one chakra, it will have an impact on the others as well. You'll begin to notice how the qualities of the different chakras are interconnected and synergistic.

SKILL VS. QUALITY

DISTINCTION
Skill vs. Quality

The qualities of a strong and open chakra are not skills that you have to learn; they are innate qualities that will naturally express themselves as you remove the interference to your soul's expression. A skill is something that is not innate but must be learned. A quality is something that is innate and cannot be learned, but only allowed or disallowed. This is an important distinction to see. For example, learning to play baseball is a skill. Nobody is born knowing how to hit a ball with a bat or throw and catch a ball. But with practice, the skills of baseball can be learned. But what allows a person to learn the skills of baseball are innate qualities of soul, such as fearless trying and improving and the joy of play and cooperation.

Pulling out the chair
Beneath your mind
And watching you fall upon God–
What else is there for Hafiz to do
That is any fun in this world!
– Hafiz

With that as a foundation, let's get to know our chakras!

14

FIRST CHAKRA

· ·

Name	Root Chakra.
Element	Earth.
Location	At the base of the spine just below the tail bone, halfway between the sexual organ and the anus.
Color	Bright red when healthy; burnt amber when not healthy.
Deals with	Survival, safety, security.
Blocked by	Fear, insecurity.
Physical Body Systems Supported	Feet, legs, hips, lower back, rectum, bones, spine, bone marrow, immune system, adrenal glands.
Physical Symptoms When Weakened/Blocked	Eating disorders, adrenal fatigue, problems with feet, legs, or tailbone, rectal or colon problems, spinal problems, immune disorders, osteoporosis and bone disorders.

THE QUALITIES AND REALIZATIONS OF PEOPLE WITH AN OPEN AND STRONG FIRST CHAKRA

People with an open and strong First Chakra will naturally see through many of the illusions around survival, safety and security.

ANALOGY
Sunrise and Light Switch Realizations

Here are some of the qualities and realizations they will naturally embody. These are innate qualities and realizations that have just been uncovered and remembered, not learned skills, techniques or coping mechanisms. A realization is more than an intellectual understanding of a principle; it is a deep knowing and seeing through direct experience. Realizations may come gradually in an incremental manner like the sunrise brightening the morning sky or they may just suddenly become so obvious and clear in a moment, like flipping on a light switch. Either way, once you really see it and know it, it will always be yours. You may temporarily forget it when you get deceived by illusions again, but your realizations will be what make the illusions more visible to you as illusions and not as reality.

This is obviously not a complete list, and you will be able to add more to your personal list the more open your First Chakra becomes. Some of the qualities and realizations of people with an open and strong First Chakra are:

74

- They feel a deep sense of well-being and security that is independent of outside circumstances. They know that all is well, no matter what.

- They are full of energy, vitality, passion, and the will to grow.

- They have a natural sense of confidence and a love for life. The confidence doesn't come from doing things they've done before (confidence in the known) but is a more general confidence that includes confidence in doing new things they've never done before (confidence in the unknown).

  DISTINCTION
  Confidence in the Known vs. Confidence in the Unknown

- They know that all experience is for growing and that life is for them, not against them. Even when they may not see how, they trust that life is supporting them in their personal journey of growth, and with enough time and perspective, everything will make sense and be seen with gratitude. This is deep and true security, independent of money, possessions, relationships, or status.

> *Why keep looking for EXIT signs in the middle of moments*
> *That didn't turn out to be quite what you'd expected?*
> *That kind of behavior keeps you searching in circles*
> *In a desert of seeming separation.*
> *Why not instead become that rogue violin*
> *Who is always singing songs of sadness and joy*
> *With the same sacred vehemence?*
> - Dreaming Bear, Baraka Kanaan

- They know that what is truly theirs cannot ever be taken away from them by anyone or anything, and that anything that can be taken away from them was never truly theirs to begin with, but was only entrusted to their care for a time. This includes everything that most people would think brings security- money, wealth, status, relationships, health and even their own bodies. It even includes their children. They realize that all of these things can, and eventually will be taken away, so they really don't own them, but rather have a temporary stewardship over whatever they have for as long as they have them.

  DISTINCTION
  What Can and Cannot Be Taken Away From You

> *Your children are not your children.*
> *They are the sons and daughters of Life's longing for itself.*
> *They come through you but not from you.*
> - Kahlil Gibran

- They are grateful for all that they have, no matter what it is or for how long it is, but they don't see their possessions as the source of their security.

If you realize that you have enough
You are truly rich.
- LAO TZU

If we believe that happiness arises only when some external condition is fulfilled, we consign ourselves to a perpetual state of discontent. For even when our expectations are fulfilled, sooner or later the little voice inside starts again, "More! More!" It is this habit, this almost mechanical fixation of the mind, that keeps us forever chasing rainbows, until at last we begin to suspect that the kingdom of heaven is within.
- EKNATH EASWAREN

- They are also generous with what they have because they know that there is always plenty of new supply that can be created as it is needed.

- They may have a little or a lot of money at any given time, but regardless of how much they have at any given time, they don't cling to it as though it were a scarce resource in limited supply that will run out and then they'll die. They realize that *they* are the scarce resource, not money.

- They understand that money is just a worldly recognition of value that they create for others and they have a relaxed confidence that comes from knowing that no matter what happens, they can always create value for others, so they can always create money. As a result, they don't stress out about the future, wondering if they'll have enough money to meet their needs and wants or if they're putting enough away for their retirement. The whole idea of retirement is seen differently. Retirement is just another phase of life from which they can continue to add value and therefore continue to create money.

- They realize that money cannot buy security, because true security cannot be purchased with money and in fact doesn't have to be purchased anyway, because it is already a given; a fact; it is just the nature of who they are as eternal souls. This knowing and living from true, innate security is in fact true wealth, and from that place of relaxed security, they can create as much money as they want.

A candle as it diminishes explains, Gathering more and more is not the way.
Burn, become light and heat and help. Melt.
– RUMI

- They don't see anything wrong with money. They realize that money is quite useful for buying stuff, but they see that buying stuff is all money is good for and that all stuff can (and eventually will) be taken away from them.

DISTINCTION
Wealth vs. Security

DISTINCTION
What Money Can Buy vs. What It Can't

- They know what can never be taken away from them and that is the source of their true security. Some of the things they know can never be taken away from them include:

  - Their ability to choose the meaning of whatever happens

  - Their connection with an infinite source of new supply that they can tap into to create what they need and want. New ideas, new possibilities, new ways of serving others and creating value for others, and thus creating money. Regardless of what the future brings, nothing can remove them from being connected to this infinite supply.

  - The already established fact that they are immortal souls having a temporary human experience, here by choice and here to experience life through their current body and personality. Even death cannot take away from them who they truly are.

  - Their knowledge that they are here to evolve and that Life is for them, not against them. That whatever happens is for their continued growth and evolution and therefore not to be feared.

- What is true of money is also true of personal relationships. Their sense of security does not come from their being in a relationship. They see being in a relationship as wonderful and something they just naturally seek out because that's what they desire, not because that's what they need to feel secure. Just as innate security is true wealth and enables the creation of all the money they need, so innate security is true love and enables them to create deep and loving relationships. They stay in relationships *from* love, instead of *for* love; in other words, love is a place they come from and bring to their relationships instead of a place they are trying to get to by being in a relationship.

DISTINCTION
Relationships For Love vs.
Relationships From Love

THE REACTIONS AND BELIEFS OF PEOPLE WITH A BLOCKED OR WEAK FIRST CHAKRA

People with a blocked and weak or compromised First Chakra cannot yet see through many of the illusions relating to survival, safety and security. As a result they will tend to react in certain ways and believe certain things to be real and those reactions and beliefs will have an impact on their physical bodies and the way they experience life. If you notice any of these reactions or beliefs to be familiar, see it as an opportunity to challenge what you may currently believe to be real. Know that as you commit to a process of daily chakra cleaning and strengthening that you will naturally begin to move away from old beliefs and reactions outlined below and towards those qualities and realizations outlined above. Some of the reactions and beliefs of people with a blocked or weak First Chakra are:

- They feel a general lack of physical energy and vitality and as a result experience a lackluster will to create.

- They live primarily from a fear-motivated sense of survival.

Fear has only two causes: the thought of losing what you have or the thought of not getting what you want.
- BYRON KATIE

- They feel a general lack of confidence, especially when dealing with the unknown.

- Life feels like a heavy struggle for survival.

- Their sense of well-being is highly dependent upon their external circumstances. So long as everything is going smoothly and to their liking, they'll feel OK, but never really great, because there is a lurking fear that their security is always under threat and that at any moment their security could be taken away from them.

- They experience frequent illness due to chronic anxiety.

- They believe that money is what creates security, and that there is some number that will guarantee their security. As a result, they see money as the scarce and powerful resource and they see themselves as weak supplicant. This results in a general sense of neediness and clinging about money.

Anybody who tries to cling to what is changing cannot help feeling insecure.
- EKNATH EASWAREN

- They treat people differently depending upon how much money they have compared to themselves. People with more money than them they treat with deference (and often jealousy) and people with less they treat with condescension or pity.

- They see relationships very much like money; as something that will make them feel secure instead of as something that naturally comes from true security. As a result, their relationships are often troubled because they are operating from an illusory mindset of neediness. "I need you to love me or my life is meaningless" is a common belief. Listen to much of the lyrics for pop music and you'll notice how pervasive this illusion is and how strong it is because of how much collective belief is given to it by humanity.

FIRST CHAKRA QUICK LIST

This is a quick summary of some of the realizations associated with an open and strong First Chakra:

- My true security is innate within me, as a part of who I really am as an eternal soul.

- All forms of external security are ultimately illusions.

- External = Temporary. Internal = Eternal.

- The unknown is a wonderful place to hang out in and nothing to be scared of.

- What is truly mine cannot be taken from me.

- Whatever can be taken from me is not truly mine and is not the source of my security.

- Money is useful for buying stuff, not freedom, security or love, which cannot be purchased, but only found within.

- Relationships are wonderful as a way of expressing and sharing love, not as a source of security and evidence that I am loveable.

- Life is for me, not against me.

- All is well.

- If I think I need something I don't have, I'm believing an illusion.

> *What sort of person says that he or she wants to be polished and pure,*
> *Then complains about being handled roughly?...*
> *The severe treatment is not toward you, but the qualities that block your growth.*
> *A rug beater doesn't beat the rug, but rather the dirt...*
> *Don't run from those who scold,*
> *And don't turn away from cleansing conflict,*
> *Or you will remain weak.*
> —RUMI

SECOND CHAKRA

Name	Sacral Chakra.
Element	Water.
Location	Lower abdomen, about two inches below the navel.
Color	Bright orange when healthy; burnt/dirty orange when not healthy.
Deals with	Pleasure, relationships, creativity, self-worth.
Blocked by	Guilt.
Physical Body Systems Supported	Reproductive organs, bowels/intestines, kidneys, bladder.
Physical Symptoms When Weakened/Blocked	Reproductive organ disorders, sexual appetite imbalances, bowel disorders, appendicitis, bladder or urinary tract problems, chronic lower back pain.

THE QUALITIES AND REALIZATIONS OF PEOPLE WITH AN OPEN AND STRONG SECOND CHAKRA

People with an open and strong Second Chakra will naturally see through many of the illusions around guilt, self-judgment and self-worth. Here are some of the qualities and realizations they will naturally embody. These are innate qualities and realizations that have just been uncovered and remembered, not learned skills, techniques or coping mechanisms. A realization is more than an intellectual understanding of a principle; it is a deep knowing and seeing through direct experience. Realizations may come gradually in an incremental manner like the sunrise brightening the morning sky or they may just suddenly become so obvious and clear in a moment, like flipping on a light switch. Either way, once you really see it and know it, it will always be yours. You may temporarily forget it when you get deceived by illusions again, but your realizations will be what make the illusions more visible to you as illusions and not as reality.

This is obviously not a complete list as you will be able to add more to your personal list the more open your Second Chakra becomes. Some of the qualities and realizations of people with an open and strong Second Chakra are:

- They feel a healthy sense of self-worth and self-esteem based on a foundation of true internal security from the First Chakra.

- As a result they are flexible and responsive to whatever life brings them; they flow like water around obstacles.

> *How can a man's life keep its course*
> *If he will not let it flow?*
> *Those who flow as life flows know*
> *They need no other force:*
> *They feel no wear, they feel no tear,*
> *They need no mending, no repair.*
> - LAO TZU

- They are self-forgiving, seeing no value in clinging to guilt over past mistakes and inconsistencies, which they actually see as learning opportunities instead of evidence of their unworthiness.

> *Don't be a searcher wrapped in the importance of his quest. Repent of your repenting!*
> - RUMI

- They realize that all forgiveness is self-forgiveness and that to forgive literally means "to give away." To give away what? The belief that they need to be punished for their mistakes and inconsistencies, either by others, or by Life or by God or by themselves.

> *It is in pardoning that we are pardoned.*
> – SAINT FRANCIS OF ASSISI

- They realize that all their past actions represent the best they could muster at the time given their then current perceptions and state of mind- regardless of what they "knew they *should* do." They see that their current perceptions are a function of their current state of mind and they realize that their state of mind is in constant flux, and not always in their total control. This realization allows them to calm and reassure the self-judging voice of their personality. When the personality accusingly scolds, "You know better than that, you're so weak! What were you thinking?", they are able to respond, "It's not what was I thinking, but what was I learning? That's a more useful question."

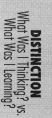
DISTINCTION
What Was I Thinking? vs.
What Was I Learning?

DISTINCTION
Consequences as Teacher vs. Judge

DISTINCTION
Forgiving vs. Nothing To Forgive

DISTINCTION
Qualified vs. Worthy

- They see that if this is true for them, it is also true for all others, so they cut themselves and others infinite slack knowing that we're all learning to uncover our souls and shine and we're all learning on our own pace and it's not their job to dictate how that should happen.

- They see the consequences of their actions as teachers, not as condemning judges declaring them unworthy.

- They come to see that the idea of needing to forgive themselves was a mistake based on an illusion that there was something to forgive in the first place. They see that true forgiveness is seeing that there was never anything to forgive in the first place, and that the consequence of not forgiving was the very punishment they thought they needed to have. (Don't worry if you find this hard to accept. You don't have to accept anything I share; just don't let that stop you from experimenting with the idea yourself and seeing what you see, allowing for the possibility of seeing it differently in the future than you have in the past.)

> *Forgiveness is discovering that what you thought happened, didn't.*
> - BYRON KATIE

- They realize the important distinction between *worthy* and *qualified*. They see that every human being is innately worthy and that worthiness cannot be earned or unearned; it can only be connected to or disconnected from. Regardless of past actions or current actions, their innate worthiness as human beings is untouchable. However, they also realize that there are many different ways in which we can be either qualified or unqualified to have or do certain things. For example, in order to practice as a medical doctor, they must first become qualified to do so by graduating from medical school. But being qualified to be a doctor is totally independent of worthiness, which is innate and untouchable.

- Like a flowing stream, they realize that they are constantly in a state of renewal. Just as you can't step in the same stream of water twice because a new supply of water has already flowed through, they realize they are not the same people today that they were yesterday. Billions of cells have been replaced in a flow much like the stream of water. They see that as human beings, our physical bodies are constantly changing, and our energy bodies are constantly changing. The only thing that can sometimes get stuck is our beliefs about how things should and should not be in order for things to be "right" in the eyes of our personality.

- They have developed strength and flexibility in both their physical bodies and in their ways of thinking and interacting with others.

- They have learned to question and drop beliefs that no longer serve them and can often become a deterrent to their staying with the natural flow of life.

- They spend the majority of their time in the receptive/flow mode of thinking, with their attention focused on doing well whatever is right in front of them to do in the moment and without getting caught in churn mode worrying about the future or overwhelming themselves with the thought of how much work there is to do.

THE REACTIONS AND BELIEFS OF PEOPLE WITH A BLOCKED OR WEAK SECOND CHAKRA

People with a blocked and weak or compromised Second Chakra cannot yet see through many of the illusions relating to guilt, self-judgment and self-worth. As a result they will tend to react in certain ways and believe certain things to be real and those reactions and beliefs will have an impact on their physical bodies and the way they experience life. If you notice any of these reactions or beliefs to be familiar, see it as an opportunity to challenge what you may currently believe to be real. Know that as you commit to a process of daily chakra cleaning and strengthening that you will naturally begin to move away from old beliefs and reactions outlined below and towards those qualities and realizations outlined above. Some of the reactions and beliefs of people with a blocked or weak Second Chakra are:

- They are often plagued by guilt and unwilling to forgive themselves, even if they manage to forgive others.

> *No particle can grow to seedling from anything but the whole.*
> *You know this. Why this continuous personal critique?*
> – RUMI

- They often have a fragile sense of self-worth and self-esteem and as a result fall into a mode of trying too hard to please others, or at least to not displease others, especially those they perceive as having power and authority over them.

- They get easily offended and feel abused or upset by the words and actions of others.

> *There is no greater misfortune*
> *Than feeling "I have an enemy";*
> *When two opponents meet,*
> *The one without an enemy*
> *Will surely triumph.*
> - LAO TZU

- They don't trust that they can be loved just for being who they already are, believing instead that they have to change themselves to become worthy of their own love, let alone the love of others.

- They often become self-sacrificing martyrs, always putting others' wants and demands before their own needs (while harboring silent resentment and grudges).

- They self-sacrifice, not out of unconditional love, but out of a craving to be accepted by others – even though they haven't ever really accepted and loved themselves first.

- They can also be very stubborn and inflexible, and this usually shows up both in their bodies and in their beliefs. They develop beliefs that are stronger than their willingness to question them and thus, when confronted with obstacles and challenges to their ways of seeing and believing, they get defensive and tend to condemn others who see things differently. When the winds of life blow, their inflexibility causes them to break rather than bend.

All things, including the grass and trees,
Are soft and pliable in life;
Dry and brittle in death.
Stiffness is thus a companion of death;
Flexibility a companion of life.
The hard and stiff will be broken;
The soft and pliable will prevail.
- LAO TZU

- They have rigid opinions and preferences and are easily upset and annoyed when anything happens that doesn't fit within their rigid preference system. They are conditioned to feel happy only so long as they get everything the way they like it, otherwise they are usually unhappy about something.

- They have a hard time distinguishing between worthiness and qualification. They often feel like their actions or their bodies or the way they were raised causes them to be unworthy. When they believe that illusion they judge and punish themselves. One of the ways they do is by avoiding situations that would put them in the company of people they see as more worthy than they are because that would just make them feel even more unworthy in comparison and they'd rather not be reminded of it. So they tend to create circles of friends that they see as more or less equal to themselves in terms of worthiness.

SECOND CHAKRA QUICK LIST

This is a quick summary of some of the realizations associated with an open and strong Second Chakra:

- My worth is innate and untouchable. It cannot be earned or unearned by my actions, it just is.

- I can be qualified or unqualified for any number of things, but none of my qualifications has anything to do with my innate worthiness.

- All forgiveness is self-forgiveness.

- To forgive is to give away the idea that you or anyone else needs to be punished for making mistakes.

- To forgive is to see through the illusion that there was something to forgive in the first place.

- Everybody is always doing the best they can given the amount of illusions they are believing at the time.

- I am in a constant state of flow and renewal and am therefore not ever bound to my past or to any particular future.

- I prefer what is and adapt and flow with it.

- I question and challenge my beliefs and drop those that no longer serve me, no matter where they came from.

- Staying in a flow state of mind is where I am happiest and accomplish the most with the least amount of effort.

- I don't know how things are going to unfold, and I prefer it that way.

And those heroic vows
No one can keep…
But still God is delighted and amused
You once tried to be a saint.
– Hafiz

16

THIRD CHAKRA

Name	Solar Plexus Chakra.
Element	Fire.
Location	Solar plexus, about two inches above the navel.
Color	Bright yellow when healthy; weak yellow/whitish/bluish when not healthy.
Deals with	Willpower, ambition, action, sense of separate personality (ego).
Blocked by	Shame, embarrassment, self-consciousness.
Physical Body Systems Supported	Liver, pancreas, gallbladder, stomach, spleen.
Physical Symptoms When Weakened/Blocked	Pancreas disorders, diabetes, hypoglycemia, digestive disorders/ulcers, liver disorders, hiatal hernias, gallstones, hemorrhoids, varicose veins, spleen problems.

THE QUALITIES AND REALIZATIONS OF PEOPLE WITH AN OPEN AND STRONG THIRD CHAKRA

People with an open and strong Third Chakra will naturally see through many of the illusions around ambition, action and accomplishment. Here are some of the qualities and realizations they will naturally embody. These are innate qualities and realizations that have just been uncovered and remembered, not learned skills, techniques or coping mechanisms. A realization is more than an intellectual understanding of a principle; it is a deep knowing and seeing through direct experience. Realizations may come gradually in an incremental manner like the sunrise brightening the morning sky or they may just suddenly become so obvious and clear in a moment, like flipping on a light switch. Either way, once you really see it and know it, it will always be yours. You may temporarily forget it when you get deceived by illusions again, but your realizations will be what make the illusions more visible to you as illusions and not as reality.

This is obviously not a complete list as you will be able to add more to your personal list the more open your Third Chakra becomes. Some of the qualities and realizations of people with an open and strong Third Chakra are:

- They have a strong sense of personal power and use it in healthy ways in the service of others.

- They are inspired to make a difference in the world, not just by dreaming, but by taking inspired action.

Serve the needs of others, and all your own needs will be fulfilled.
Through selfless action, fulfillment is attained.
- Lao Tzu

Even after all this time
The sun never says to the earth,
"You owe me."
Look what happens
With a love like that.
It lights up the whole sky
– Hafiz

- They are not overly self-conscious; they don't worry about what other people think of them. They are more interested in making a difference, and they understand that the criticism of others is likely to come with the territory of pushing past comfort zones.

- They operate in a fearless manner. Being fearless is very different from being brave or courageous. Being brave or courageous is feeling fearful and taking action anyway, often in defiance of fear. Being fearless is seeing more clearly that there is nothing to fear in the first place, that it was just an illusion. This is very similar to seeing that there was nothing to forgive in the first place.

- They feel a deep sense of purpose that they realize comes from their soul having specific things it's here to do. They are able to see and feel the distinction between what their soul is inspiring them to do and what their personality is motivating them to do (or not do).

DISTINCTION
Brave vs. Fearless

Don't ask what the world needs. Ask what makes you come alive, and go do it.
Because what the world needs is people who have come alive.
- Howard Thurman

There is one thing in this world you must never forget to do. If you forget everything else and not this, there's nothing to worry about, but if you remember everything else and forget this, then you will have done nothing in your life.
It's as if a king has sent you to some country to do a task, and you perform a hundred other services, but not the one he sent you to do. So human beings come to this world to do particular work. That work is the purpose, and each is specific to the person.
– RUMI

DISTINCTION
Dealing with Challenges vs. Creating Challenges

- They see the entire concept of failure very differently. Failure is seen as necessary and even desirable. It is evidence that they are getting out of their comfort zones and voluntarily challenging themselves because they know that is the best and most painless way to grow.

Then the time came when the risk it took to remain tight in a bud was more painful than the risk it took to blossom.
- ANAIS NIN

ANALOGY
Facing Challenges; Lifting Weights

- They see challenges as something that benefits them instead of an affront to the comfortable life they have somehow earned or deserve, sort of like lifting weights helps them increase their strength and power. In a way, they have become like little children again. Little children thrive on challenge. They invent ways of challenging themselves when they don't feel challenged enough, because they know that's where the real fun is. "Look, Ma – no hands!" They don't just deal with challenges as an inevitable part of living, but they create challenges by pursuing dreams.

To grow to our full height, we need to be challenged with tasks that draw out our deeper resources, the talents and capacities we did not know we had. We need to be faced with obstacles that cannot be surmounted unless we summon up our daring and creativity. This kind of challenge is familiar to any great athlete or scientist or artist. No worthwhile accomplishment comes easily.
-EKNATH EASWAREN

- They thrive on doing things they've never done before and like to always have something to be involved in that takes them into the unknown and uncomfortable.

DISTINCTION
Motivated Action vs. Inspired Action

- They see a clear distinction between motivated action and inspired action. Motivated action is action that is motivated by the personality in an attempt to make it feel more secure. Inspired action is action that is prompted by the soul's innate desire to express its true nature. Such action is often resisted by the personality because it may involve taking the personality out of its well-protected safety zone.

When you do things from your soul, you feel a river moving in you, a joy.
When actions come from another section, the feeling disappears.
Don't let others lead you. They may be blind or, worse, vultures.
Reach for the rope of God. And what is that?
Putting aside self-will…
If you could leave your selfishness,
You would see how you've been torturing your soul…
Don't insist on going where your think you want to go.
Ask the way to the spring.
— RUMI

- They don't get paralyzed about making decisions that seem big to others. Instead they see decisions as just motion in a particular direction that will guarantee them more information than they had before making the decision. With that new information, they can make a different decision and keep moving in a new direction. They see that there are very few irreversible or unalterable decisions in life, so they are fearless about making decisions and learning what there is to learn from having made that decision.

DISTINCTION Decisions=Motion+Info vs. Decisions=Less Freedom

No one knows for certain
Whether the vessel will sink or reach the harbor.
Cautious people say,
"I'll do nothing until I can be sure."
Merchants know better.
If you do nothing, you lose.
Don't be one of those merchants who won't risk the ocean!
This is much more important than losing or making money.
This is your connection to God.
You must set fire to have light.
Trust means you're ready to risk what you currently have.
— RUMI

- They are clear on the distinction between being highly engaged in action vs. highly attached to the outcome. They stay highly engaged in doing well what needs to be done in the moment, keeping their attention focused in the present moment, on the task at hand. At the same time, they are not highly attached to the outcome of whatever they are working on, meaning that their sense of security, worth and well-being are not attached to how any particular project or decision turns out. They care about results, and adapt their actions if they don't seem to be leading to the desired results, but they keep their attention focused on what is within their control.

DISTINCTION Highly Engaged vs. Highly Attached

The master can keep giving
Because there is no end to his wealth,
He acts without expectation,
Succeeds without taking credit,
And does not think that he is better
Than anyone else.
- LAO TZU

- They are contribution minded instead of accomplishment minded. They don't need accomplishments to prove anything to themselves or anyone else. They see that personal accomplishment is a pursuit of the personality, not the soul. Instead they are inspired to contribute whatever they feel driven to contribute to others. They can always control what they contribute and they get deep satisfaction out of contributing to the best of their ability, regardless of how others accept it or how other factors outside of their control affect the outcome.

One with true virtue always seeks to give.
One who lacks true virtue always seeks a way to get.
To the giver, comes the fullness of life;
To the taker, just an empty hand.
- LAO TZU

- They have a healthy and balanced appetite and metabolism. They are drawn to naturally healthy foods because they are sensitive to the impact of the quality of foods on the energy of all three bodies (physical, energy, and spirit).

THE REACTIONS AND BELIEFS OF PEOPLE WITH A BLOCKED OR WEAK THIRD CHAKRA

People with a blocked and weak or compromised Third Chakra cannot yet see through many of the illusions relating to ambition, action and accomplishment. As a result they will tend to react in certain ways and believe certain things to be real and those reactions and beliefs will have an impact on their physical bodies and the way they experience life. If you notice any of these reactions or beliefs to be familiar, see it as an opportunity to challenge what you may currently believe to be real. Know that as you commit to a process of daily chakra cleaning and strengthening that you will naturally begin to move away from old beliefs and reactions outlined below and towards those qualities and realizations outlined above. Some of the reactions and beliefs of people with a blocked or weak Third Chakra are:

- They see their world primarily through a filter of fear and anxiety.

- They see themselves as victims of circumstances and the decisions of other people.

- They see themselves as powerless relative to some people and powerful relative to others. For example, this may show up in being overly submissive at work while being a tyrant at home.

- They often give their personal power away to others because they are fearful of creating an uncomfortable confrontation.

- They are highly self-conscious, meaning they are always wondering what any event or possible outcome in the future will say about them, or what others will think of them. "If I try this and it fails, what will that say about me?" is a question that dominates their decision making.

What People May Think
Some people cower
And wince and shrink,
Owing to the fear of
What people may think.
There is one answer
To worries like these:
People may think
What the devil they please.
-PIET HIEN

- They are easily embarrassed and frequently beat themselves up with their own thinking.

- They have lots of different ways of shaming themselves.

- The prospect of trying and failing isn't nearly as fearful as the prospect of looking like a failure to others.

- Fear and anxiety are frequent companions. The future is viewed as full of danger and threat, and so they are constantly in a state of playing it safe.

- They don't trust their ability to adapt and overcome anything that comes their way.

- They are very sensitive to stress and often think about and talk about how stressful their lives are and how stressed-out they feel.

- A physical body sign of a weak Third Chakra is an unbalanced appetite: either very weak or very strong.

THIRD CHAKRA QUICK LIST

This is a quick summary of some of the realizations associated with an open and strong Third Chakra:

- I'm here to contribute and serve, not out-accomplish others.

- I am the owner and author of my life's experience, not a victim of anyone or anything.

- Fearless is seeing through the illusion of fear.

- If I'm not failing occasionally, I'm avoiding growth.

- Decisions are just motion in a particular direction that always provides more information than I had before. I can always make a new decision based on new information.

- Inspired action only. Is this coming from my soul wanting to express itself and contribute or is it coming from my personality wanting to feel more secure?

- High engagement, low attachment = enjoyment and peace.

It is natural to feel that a little status or recognition would not be unwelcome in addition to earning a good livelihood, yet all the world's great religions teach us that getting something out of life, whether it is money or recognition or power or prestige, is not our real need. Giving to life is our real need.
    – Eknath Easwaren

FOURTH CHAKRA

Name	Heart Chakra.
Element	Love.
Location	Center of ribs at heart level.
Color	Bright green when healthy; dark/dirty green when not healthy.
Deals with	Love, compassion, belonging.
Blocked by	Grief, clinging, loneliness.
Physical Body Systems Supported	Heart, lungs, chest, arteries/veins, upper back, shoulders, arms, and hands.
Physical Symptoms When Weakened/Blocked	Heart disorders: heart attacks, congestive heart failure, valve problems, chest pain, arteriosclerosis, peripheral vascular insufficiency. Also asthma, allergies, lung disorders, pneumonia, bronchitis, emphysema, breast lumps/cysts, circulation problems, tension or pain between shoulder blades; shoulder, arm, and hand problems like carpal tunnel.

THE QUALITIES AND REALIZATIONS OF PEOPLE WITH AN OPEN AND STRONG FOURTH CHAKRA

People with an open and strong Fourth Chakra will naturally see through many of the illusions around love, compassion, grief, loneliness and belonging. Here are some of the qualities and realizations they will naturally embody. These are innate qualities and realizations that have just been uncovered and remembered, not learned skills, techniques or coping mechanisms. A realization is more than an intellectual understanding of a principle; it is a deep knowing and seeing through direct experience. Realizations may come gradually in an incremental manner like the sunrise brightening the morning sky or they may just suddenly become so obvious and clear in a moment, like flipping on a light switch. Either way, once you really see it and know it, it will always be yours. You may temporarily forget it when you get deceived by illusions again, but your realizations will be what make the illusions more visible to you as illusions and not as reality.

This is obviously not a complete list as you will be able to add more to your personal list the more open your Fourth Chakra becomes. Some of the qualities and realizations of people with an open and strong Fourth Chakra are:

- They are naturally loving, compassionate, and understanding of self and others.

- They are seen as warm, friendly, and approachable.

Love makes everything that is heavy, light.
– THOMAS A KEMPIS

DISTINCTION
Judging with Condemnation vs. Judging with Compassion

- They realize that exercising judgment is not something to be avoided but that when judgments are made, there are essentially two choices: condemnation or compassion. The more open and healthy the Fourth Chakra, the more natural it becomes to choose compassion; condemnation doesn't even make logical sense any more, let alone feel right. Their thinking would go something like this:

"How could I possibly know everything that person is dealing with—all their past conditioning, beliefs, and assumptions? I don't even really understand my own behavior much of the time, so why would I presume to understand theirs? All I know is that it's very easy to get caught up in my own thinking and automatically believe my thinking to be true. It certainly feels true at the time, and when I believe it to be true, even though it is often an illusion I am believing, I often act based on that belief, and my actions make things worse instead of better. If I know that happens to me when I'm in a lower state of mind, why would I expect it to be any different for anyone else? If anything, this person may be less aware than I am of how easy it is to get deceived by your own thinking and I have compassion for them and feel even more connected to them as a fellow human being."

But charity means pardoning what is unpardonable, or it is no virtue at all. Hope means hoping when things are hopeless, or it is no virtue at all. And faith means believing the incredible, or it is no virtue at all.
– G. K. CHESTERTON

- They are natural peacemakers. They don't get caught up in escalating arguments because they don't have an intense need to be right.

Don't try to figure this out.
Love's work looks absurd,
But trying to find a meaning
Will hide it more. Silence.
– RUMI

- They are great listeners. They listen to others in a natural, compassionate way without the need to agree, disagree, or analyze what the others are saying. They listen to others more like they listen to beautiful music – for the pure enjoyment of it. They listen for meaning, not necessarily content. Listening for meaning is listening with the intent to really feel what the other person means, even if they aren't saying it in words, or their words even mask or contradict what they are really feeling. Because their attention is focused completely on the other person and not distracted by their own worries and self-consciousness, they are open to feeling in their heart what is really being communicated below the verbal level.

  DISTINCTION
  Listening for Content vs.
  Listening for Meaning

- Their words and responses go beyond feeling the other person's pain and sympathizing with it. They go beyond sympathy and compassion for the other person and offer calm and peaceful reassurance. They can see that the insecurity and suffering is coming from the other person's personality and they have compassion for that while at the same time knowing that the other person also has a soul and can find their own peace and answers. Even without needing to explain it in those terms, this knowing helps to settle the agitated, anxious and fearful state of mind of the other. The reassurance isn't that everything will always work out the way the personality wants it to, but that everything will always work out the way that will lead to their continued evolution even if that means some temporary pain the personality has to go through to stop resisting and start allowing.

  DISTINCTION
  Sympathy vs. Reassurance

For all I care about
Is quenching your thirst for freedom!
All a Sane man can ever care about
Is giving Love!
– HAFIZ

If emotions were made of chocolate, some of the darkest ones would surely taste the best.
- DREAMING BEAR, BARAKA KANAAN

- They feel connected to and harmonious with all creation: other people, animals, nature, and the universe at large.

- They have radiating or glowing countenances and bright, clear eyes.

DISTINCTION
Resisting vs. Allowing vs. Loving What Is

- They come from a place of loving what is, instead of resisting what is. This doesn't mean they are not inspired to take action to improve things that are within their power. The opposite is actually true: they are masters at doing that. It just means that the actions they take are coming from a place of acceptance and even an embracing of what is, rather than of resistance. This allows them to have greater access to the wisdom, creativity, and insight that will actually help them change things in the most effective way possible. Author, speaker, and teacher Byron Katie (www.byronkatie.com) is to me one of the most powerfully loving people I have ever met. I have no doubt that her Fourth Chakra is wide open and radiating brightly. I could literally feel it in her presence. I highly recommend her work to all and utilize it in the coaching work I do with clients.

Woman with Flower

I wouldn't coax the plant if I were you.
Such watchful nurturing may do it harm.
Let the soil rest from so much digging
And wait until it's dry before you water it.
The leaf's inclined to find its own direction;
Give it a chance to seek the sunlight for itself.
Much growth is stundted by too careful prodding,
Too eager tenderness.
The things we love we have to learn to leave alone.
-Naomi Long Madgett

- They realize that they are never upset for the reasons they think they are upset. If they are upset, it is not because of some external circumstance, but because they are seeing something that isn't there- they are seeing an illusion.

DISTINCTION
Desires of the Personality vs. Desires of the Soul

- They live contented lives. They have stepped off the treadmill of personality discontentment, of always wanting more; more money, more control, more respect of others, or more accomplishment. They are clear on the distinction between the desires of the soul and the desires of the personality. As a result, they can distinguish between a discontented soul that drives them to greater levels of awareness and love and a discontented personality that drives them to greater levels of accomplishment and recognition.

There is no greater loss than losing the Tao,
No greater curse than covetousness,
No greater tragedy than discontentment;
The worst of faults is wanting more- always.
Contentment alone is enough.
Indeed, the bliss of eternity
Can be found in your contentment.
- Lao Tzu

THE REACTIONS AND BELIEFS OF PEOPLE WITH A BLOCKED OR WEAK FOURTH CHAKRA

People with a blocked and weak or compromised Fourth Chakra cannot yet see through many of the illusions relating to love, compassion, grief, loneliness and belonging. As a result they will tend to react in certain ways and believe certain things to be real and those reactions and beliefs will have an impact on their physical bodies and the way they experience life. If you notice any of these reactions or beliefs to be familiar, see it as an opportunity to challenge what you may currently believe to be real. Know that as you commit to a process of daily chakra cleaning and strengthening that you will naturally begin to move away from old beliefs and reactions outlined below and towards those qualities and realizations outlined above. Some of the reactions and beliefs of people with a blocked or weak Fourth Chakra are:

- They are often guarded and closed. They may have been hurt by ones they loved in the past and developed a belief that they must always be on guard against getting hurt again, so they never really allow themselves to get close to others.

- They are highly judgmental and condemning of themselves and others, looking to find and assign fault wherever something doesn't go the way they think it should. In fact, they are often unable to let a situation rest until they have assigned fault and blame to all people they see as responsible for things not going the way they wanted them to go.

How can we live in harmony?
First we need to know
We are all madly in love
With the same God
- Thomas Aquinas

- They assign motive to everything anyone does that impacts them. They are sure that the motive they assigned is actually correct, not seeing (yet) that they couldn't possibly know.

- "Mercy for me, justice for you" is a common mindset. I call this the Jonah syndrome, referring to the Old Testament prophet Jonah who was cast overboard during a brutal storm at sea but then swallowed by a whale and preserved and given another chance to do what he had originally run away from. He prayed for and received mercy, but then when the people of Tarsus, who were enemies to the Israelites, listened to him and repented and changed their ways, Jonah wasn't happy about the mercy they received, and was instead angry at God for not destroying them. He wanted justice for them, but was fine accepting mercy for himself.

- They are easily offended and upset by the words and actions of others that do not conform to their view of how things should be.

- They resist what is if they don't like it and then often take personality based action to try to fix it to be more to their liking.

> God is trying to sell you something
> But you don't want to buy.
> That is what your suffering is;
> Your fantastic haggling
> Your manic screaming over the price!
> – HAFIZ

- Their personal relationships are based on needing the other person to love them so they can return the love. This means their love is always conditioned upon the other person conforming to their expectations. As long as they do, all is well. As soon as they don't, big problem!

> Seeking love keeps you from the awareness that you already are it.
> - BYRON KATIE

- They see the need to fix other people and often try to do so. They become clingy and needy, and as a result often end up lonely and grieving the loss of love, which they always see as something they have to find outside themselves.

- No matter how much wealth or recognition they have, they are never content for very long. They seem unable to get off the treadmill of always wanting more.

FOURTH CHAKRA QUICK LIST

This is a quick summary of some of the realizations associated with an open and strong Fourth Chakra:

- If I judge, I judge with compassion, both for myself and for others

- I listen to others for meaning, not just content. I have nothing on my mind when listening to others, that way I am open to feeling what they really mean to say even if they don't say it with words.

- What we all want when we're feeling insecure is reassurance, not sympathy or agreement.

- Action that comes from resisting what is, just causes more resistance. Accept, embrace and love what is and then act from there, if action still makes sense, which often it doesn't.

- Mercy for me. Mercy for you.

- I don't need you to love me in order for me to love me.

- I don't need to and can't fix anyone. I can only strengthen my own connection to my soul and be an example to others and assist them to do the same.

- No one is ever lost, not even in death. We are all connected.

Let's stop reading about God–
We will never understand Him.
Jump to your feet, wave your fists,
Threaten and warn the whole Universe
That your heart can no longer live
Without real love!
– Hafiz

18

FIFTH CHAKRA

Name	Throat Chakra.
Element	Sound.
Location	Center of throat.
Color	Light blue when healthy; blue/gray when not healthy.
Deals with	Truth, expression, communication.
Blocked by	Lies, especially the ones we tell ourselves.
Physical Body Systems Supported	Neck, jaw, teeth, gums, mouth, lower sinus, throat, thyroid.
Physical Symptoms When Weakened/Blocked	Jaw problems, TMJ, swollen glands in the throat, neck problems, chronic childhood tonsillitis, thyroid disorders, chronic sinus problems; disorders of the throat, mouth, teeth, or gums.

THE QUALITIES AND REALIZATIONS OF PEOPLE WITH AN OPEN AND STRONG FIFTH CHAKRA

People with an open and strong Fifth Chakra will naturally see through many of the illusions around honesty, integrity, expression and communication. Here are some of the qualities and realizations they will naturally embody. These are innate qualities and realizations that have just been uncovered and remembered, not learned skills, techniques or coping mechanisms. A realization is more than an intellectual understanding of a principle; it is a deep knowing and seeing through direct experience. Realizations may come gradually in an incremental manner like the sunrise brightening the morning sky or they may just suddenly become so obvious and clear in a moment, like flipping on a light switch. Either way, once you really see it and know it, it will always be yours. You may temporarily forget it when you get deceived by illusions again, but your realizations will be what make the illusions more visible to you as illusions and not as reality.

This is obviously not a complete list as you will be able to add more to your personal list the more open your Fifth Chakra becomes. Some of the qualities and realizations of people with an open and strong Fifth Chakra are:

- They naturally exhibit both an open mind and an open heart. As a result, they speak their truth with authenticity, clarity and confidence.

> *You are the truth*
> *From foot to brow.*
> *Now, what else would you like to know?*
> – RUMI

- They also face the truth without trying to avoid it or hide from it. They are not afraid of the truth. The truth is *always* their friend, even if it requires going through some discomfort or challenge for the personality.

> *Truth is such an understanding lover,*
> *Infinitely patient and kind…*
> *She always keeps her bedroom window cracked open,*
> *Incase you suddenly develop the courage in the middle of the night,*
> *To climb in and curl up close to her covers of compassion.*
> - DREAMING BEAR, BARAKA KANAAN

- They like to share their positive vision with others and see it as speaking their desire into reality. They are not afraid to make specific requests of others to help them bring about their desires. They enjoy enrolling others in the process of creating what they want to create by helping them see how their getting involved will benefit themselves and others.

> *Why keep your divine gifts locked away in a dark room of neglect*
> *Half-starved from being unshared.*
> *Don't you know dreams die like that?*
> - DREAMING BEAR, BARAKA KANAAN

- They know that if they don't ask, the answer is always no. They are not fazed by being told "no." They don't see it as a rejection of themselves, but rather just another form of truth, which is always their friend. Either their request was not the right fit now for this particular person or it wasn't creative enough to really engage the other person. In either case, there is more clarity and a new decision can be made from a place of greater clarity.

- They see the distinction between surface truth and deep truth and they speak deep truth. Surface appearances are often not the truth at all, but rather the illusion.

DISTINCTION
No= Rejection vs. No=Truth

DISTINCTION
Surface Truth vs. Deep Truth

Deep truth is truth that may not be obvious on the surface, but they know is there underneath. They see the deep truth that everyone they deal with is in fact a divine soul having a human experience, just like they are. This shows up in how they treat and speak to people who are caught up in their own stressful thinking and reacting in a self-defeating way. Their words are calming and reassuring.

> *The great leader speaks little.*
> *He never speaks carelessly.*
> *He works without self-interest*
> *And leaves no trace.*
> *When all is finished, the people say,*
> *"We did it ourselves."*
> - LAO TZU

THE REACTIONS AND BELIEFS OF PEOPLE WITH A BLOCKED OR WEAK FIFTH CHAKRA

People with a blocked and weak or compromised Fifth Chakra cannot yet see through many of the illusions related to honesty, integrity, expression and communication. As a result they will tend to react in certain ways and believe certain things to be real and those reactions and beliefs will have an impact on their physical bodies and the way they experience life. If you notice any of these reactions or beliefs to be familiar, see it as an opportunity to challenge what you may currently believe to be real. Know that as you commit to a process of daily chakra cleaning and strengthening that you will naturally begin to move away from old beliefs and reactions outlined below and towards those qualities and realizations outlined above. Some of the reactions and beliefs of people with a blocked or weak Fifth Chakra are:

- They are afraid to speak up and say what they think.

- They tend to go along with the crowd to avoid rocking the boat.

- They don't believe that their opinions are valuable and worry that others think their opinions aren't interesting.

- They are constantly swallowing their words and may suffer from frequent sore throats and coughs.

- Not only do they rarely speak their truth to others, they often avoid facing the truth themselves. They don't trust that they are strong enough to deal with it effectively.

- They find it difficult to ask for others' assistance in helping them create their dreams.

- They tell themselves no in order to avoid the possibility that by asking others, they will be rejected.

- They see a no from others as a direct rejection of themselves as a person. This commonly shows up in a fear and loathing of selling.

- They mistake surface appearances for truth, not seeing the deeper truth that lies beneath the surface, which may be the exact opposite of the way things appear.

- They have feelings of emptiness of spirit. This emptiness often drives them to fill the void with the pursuit of riches and recognition.

FIFTH CHAKRA QUICK LIST

This is a quick summary of some of the realizations associated with an open and strong Fifth Chakra:

- Not only is it easier, but it's more powerful to be authentic then to try to impress others.

- The truth is always my friend. The truth is always kinder than the illusion.

- If I don't ask, the answer is always no.

- When I do ask and get a no or an objection, it is not a rejection of me, but another form of truth, which is always my friend and always kinder than the illusion.

- Seeing and speaking deep truth is seeing and speaking from soul to soul. Seeing and speaking surface truth is speaking from personality to personality.

There's a town where the soul is fed, where love hears truth and thrives.
And another town that produces lies that degrade and starve love.
Your voice is a small market set between the two towns.
– RUMI

19

SIXTH CHAKRA

Name	Third Eye Chakra.
Element	Thought.
Location	Center of brow, midline between eyes.
Color	Dark blue/indigo when healthy; muddy dark blue when not healthy.
Deals with	Insight, intuition, wisdom.
Blocked by	Illusions.
Physical Body Systems Supported	Upper frontal sinuses, eyes, ears, outer brain.
Physical Symptoms When Weakened/Blocked	Frequent headaches, upper/frontal sinus conditions, neurological disorders, eye disorders, glaucoma, cataracts, macular degeneration, strokes, disorders of the outer brain.

THE QUALITIES AND REALIZATIONS OF PEOPLE WITH AN OPEN AND STRONG SIXTH CHAKRA

People with an open and strong Sixth Chakra will naturally see through illusions into deeper truth. Here are some of the qualities and realizations they will naturally embody. These are innate qualities and realizations that have just been uncovered and remembered, not learned skills, techniques or coping mechanisms. A realization is more than an intellectual understanding of a principle; it is a deep knowing and seeing through direct experience. Realizations may come gradually in an incremental manner like the sunrise brightening the morning sky or they may just suddenly become so obvious and clear in a moment, like flipping on a light switch. Either way, once you really see it and know it, it will always be yours. You may temporarily forget it when you get deceived by illusions again, but your realizations will be what make the illusions more visible to you as illusions and not as reality.

This is obviously not a complete list as you will be able to add more to your personal list the more open your Sixth Chakra becomes. Some of the qualities and realizations of people with an open and strong Sixth Chakra are:

- They have a strong sense of their own inner truth. They trust and follow their own inner guidance, even in the face of their own insecure thinking or the opinions of others.

The master observes the world
But trusts his inner vision.
He allows things to come and go.
He prefers what is within to what is without.
- LAO TZU

- They are very imaginative and have a strong sense of internal vision. They are often seen and heralded as visionaries by others, but usually only after their inner vision is proved right.

- They have a strong sense of being connected to God, to life, and to all others.

Everyone is God speaking.
Why not be polite and listen to Him?
- HAFIZ

- They see life with great clarity, which allows them to live with peace and calm even amid great uncertainty.

- They realize the distinction between certainty and clarity and they seek clarity over certainty. They see that certainty is a false conclusion the personality creates to feel safe with what is unknown and maybe even unknowable. They see that all the certainties that our personalities adopt are the source of all conflict – internally, interpersonally, and between classes and nations. They see how the personality is so certain of its illusions that it doesn't seek to see through them, but defends them and condemns anyone who doesn't see things the same way. They see that "I don't know. I don't truly understand anything" is the entry way into greater clarity and that clarity exists without the need for certainty.

DISTINCTION
Certainty vs. Clarity

- They are able to recognize the role of thought as the instantaneous creator of their experience of life in the moment. They live their lives from the inside out, not the outside in. This is a fundamental shift in awareness that transforms how they see everything.

- They are able to live with most of their attention in the present moment, flowing and responding to life with wisdom and ease. As a result, they experience the simple joys of being fully present and aware of the many miracles that make up each moment.

- They experience many "MMMM" moments throughout each day. This is my name I came up with to describe the experience of seeing through a surface illusion and into the "<u>m</u>agic and <u>m</u>ystery of this <u>m</u>agnificent <u>m</u>oment" where all you can utter is "MMMM" because the depth of your perceptions cannot be put into words.

- They are comfortable in a state of not knowing; they realize that surrendering their need to know is what opens them up to receive guidance for their next steps.

Very little grows on jagged rock. Be ground.
Be crumbled so wildflowers will come up where you are.
You've been stony for too many years.
Try something different. Surrender.
— RUMI

- They don't have to know how things will turn out. They trust that by following their inner guidance a step at a time, things will turn out best for themselves and for all others.

When they think that they know the answers,
People are difficult to guide
When they know they do not know,
People can find their own way.
- LAW TZU

- They often experience heightened sensory perception, sometimes called a sixth sense. This shows up in an ability to discern what's really going on beneath the surface of appearances.

- They are able to see right to the heart of a situation and offer needed help to others. The help they offer is not in the form of bailing others out or solving their problems for them, but rather in the form of helping them see their situations with more clarity, reassuring them and reminding them of their own innate abilities to deal gracefully with whatever is happening. They make excellent coaches and teachers.

Until you see the world as innocent,
you haven't realized your own innocence.
- BYRON KATIE

- They are patient, waiting calmly for things to unfold as they will, trusting that there is a much bigger picture to life and that life is for them, not against them.

- They know that things will turn out for the best, and that doesn't necessarily need to look the way they think it should. They are able to see the wisdom in how things do turn out.

- It's not so much what they see, but what they see *with*. They see with the eyes of their souls as much as with the eyes in their heads; and if there were ever a conflict, they would trust the eyes of their souls.

DISTINCTION
What You See vs. What You See With

Do you want to act differently?
That's not possible until you perceive differently
- BYRON KATIE

If you want to see the beloved's face,
borrow the beloved's eyes.
Look through them and you'll see the face everywhere.
– RUMI

- They can look at everything good that has happened to them, and trace it back to something in the past that seemed bad at the time. This gives them added perspective. When things happen that might seem bad, they know that it is planting the seed for something great to come into their lives.

DISTINCTION
Good & Bad vs. All Good

Bad fortune is what good fortune leans on;
Good fortune is what bad fortune hides in.
Who knows the ultimate end of this process?
- LAO TZU

- They are grateful for *all* things, not just things that appear good at the moment.

He who feels punctured
Must once have been a bubble.
He who feels unarmed,
Must have carried arms.
He who feels deprived
Must have had privilege.
- LAO TZU

THE REACTIONS AND BELIEFS OF PEOPLE WITH A BLOCKED OR WEAK SIXTH CHAKRA

People with a blocked and weak or compromised Sixth Chakra cannot yet see through many illusions into deeper truth. As a result they will tend to react in certain ways and believe certain things to be real and those reactions and beliefs will have an impact on their physical bodies and the way they experience life. If you notice any of these reactions or beliefs to be familiar, see it as an opportunity to challenge what you may currently believe to be real. Know that as you commit to a process of daily chakra cleaning and strengthening that you will naturally begin to move away from old beliefs and reactions outlined below and towards those qualities and realizations outlined above. Some of the reactions and beliefs of people with a blocked or weak Sixth Chakra are:

- They have a weak connection with their own inner truth and guidance. They feel lost when it comes to a sense of purpose and a path in life. This sense of being lost can often lead to becoming very ritualistic and dogmatic in following a particular leader or system that gives them a sense of purpose or meaning.

> *When the Tao is lost, there is goodness.*
> *When goodness is lost, there is morality.*
> *When morality is lost, there is ritual.*
> *Ritual is the husk of true faith,*
> *The beginning of chaos.*
> - LAO TZU

- Their imaginations are often misused to create resentment and shame over the past, embarrassment in the present, and anxiety and worry about the future.

- They feel disconnected and alone, and they experience life as confusing and frustrating. All of this is really an illusion, but they spend most of their time with their analytical minds spinning in churn mode, trying to figure everything out and getting really frustrated when they can't, not yet seeing that they are trying to fix an illusion.

- They get caught up in their personality's insecure thinking, and as a result become highly reactive to comments of others or external conditions. This shows up in their being very snippy, getting easily annoyed or upset, and reacting with anger and self-righteous, condemning judgment of others.

- True peace of mind is a rare state for them because they are often stuck in churn mode. Temporary respites from their overactive analytical and critical thinking are usually induced by ingested substances like alcohol or drugs (both prescription and illegal) that temporarily help them ease off the gas of their revved up critical thinking and relax for a while.

- They have a difficult time translating ideas into action and are easily distracted.

- They get stuck in the constantly seeking answers mode. They may travel far and wide looking for experiences in the outside world to give them a sense of meaning and stimulation, all the while neglecting to explore within.

> *There are many going afar to marvel at the heights of mountains,*
> *the mighty waves of the sea,*
> *the long courses of great rivers, the vastness of the ocean,*
> *the movements of the stars,*
> *yet they leave themselves unnoticed!*
> – Saint Augustine

- They are rarely very present in the moment because their thinking is often stuck in churn mode; reliving past moments, analyzing them for mistakes and generating resentment and guilt, or trying desperately to figure out and be prepared for all possible contingencies in the future. As a result, they experience very little joy in the present moment.

- They have difficulty recognizing their own thinking and its impact on their experience of life. Their thinking is usually invisible to them. As a result, they believe that their experience of life is caused by outside forces, people, and circumstances.

- They tend to analyze and overanalyze how they can control circumstances to be more to their liking.

- It is difficult for them to become highly engaged in any activity because their busy, churning minds don't allow them to keep much of their attention in the moment.

- They are often highly attached to things turning out the way they want them to or think they should, so life is experienced as a constant emotional roller coaster. They feel up when things seem to be going their way, and down when things don't seem to be going their way.

The Mind is addicted to forms and worrying about things
Over which it has not control
While the Soul can be found tugging on the Heart's shirt sleeve
To whisper this secret in your ear;
There is an undiscovered universe in here.
But the Mind doesn't listen, only tears itself apart
Searching for tangible tenderness in imaginary truths.
- DREAMING BEAR, BARAKA KANAAN

SIXTH CHAKRA QUICK LIST

This is a quick summary of some of the realizations associated with an open and strong Sixth Chakra:

- My experience of life is caused 100% by my perceptions; by how clearly I see through illusion and into truth.

- I don't know how things are going to unfold and I prefer it that way.

- My personality holds many certainties that keep me from clarity.

- The more humble I am willing to be; to see that I don't see, to understand that I don't understand, to realize that I don't realize, the more clearly I will be able to see through illusions.

- I have access to all the guidance I will ever need to see through any illusions.

- The only place my attention has any power is in the present.

- Worry, anxiety, shame and regret are just misuses of imagination. My imagination is meant for higher uses.

- Anything that upsets me is a sign that I am still seeing an illusion, still seeing through the eyes of my personality, not the eyes of my soul.

- It is never anything outside me that upsets me. It is not what I see so much as what I see with.

- My work is not to control my circumstances or even my thoughts; it is to see through illusions. That is a lifetime of fascinating and fulfilling work.

- Every single circumstance or happening in my life is just another opportunity for me to practice seeing through illusions and therefore I am grateful for *all* things, not just the things that appear good to my personality.

- The most powerful way I can serve others is to help them see that they themselves have the power to see through their own illusions to the deeper truth that exists before and after all illusions.

SEVENTH CHAKRA

Name	Crown Chakra.
Element	Light/spirit.
Location	Crown of head.
Color	Bright violet/purple when healthy; muddy/dark purple when not healthy.
Deals with	Pure energy, union with divine.
Blocked by	Earthly attachments.
Physical Body Systems Supported	Deeper brain and central nervous system.
Physical Symptoms When Weakened/Blocked	Anxiety and depression disorders, bipolar disorder, migraines, amnesia, epilepsy, multiple sclerosis, Parkinson's disease, attention deficit disorders, dyslexia, ALS, cognitive delusions, mental illness.

THE QUALITIES AND REALIZATIONS OF PEOPLE WITH AN OPEN AND STRONG SEVENTH CHAKRA

People with an open and strong Seventh Chakra will naturally see through illusions related to earthly attachments and separation. Here are some of the qualities and realizations they will naturally embody. These are innate qualities and realizations that have just been uncovered and remembered, not learned skills, techniques or coping mechanisms. A realization is more than an intellectual understanding of a principle; it is a deep knowing and seeing through direct experience. Realizations may come gradually in an incremental manner like the sunrise brightening the morning sky or they may just suddenly become so obvious and clear in a moment, like flipping on a light switch. Either way, once you really see it and know it, it will always be yours. You may temporarily forget it when you get deceived by illusions again, but your realizations will be what make the illusions more visible to you as illusions and not as reality.

This is obviously not a complete list as you will be able to add more to your personal list the more open your Seventh Chakra becomes. Some of the qualities and realizations of people with an open and strong Seventh Chakra are:

- They have a powerful sense of the unity of all life and the illusion of separateness.

- They see themselves in all others and all others in themselves. This allows them to learn from anyone and everything: all people and all circumstances are their teachers. The child, the homeless person, the tree, the river, the celebrity, the criminal, the traffic, the weather – all are reflections of some aspect of themselves and are thus teachers.

> *The certainty of each other's equality will ultimately set us free.*
> - Dreaming-Bear, Baraka Kanaan

- They exhibit a natural, unbounded and unconditional love and compassion for all, not because it's the right thing to do, but because it's the only way of being that makes any sense at all.

- The pull of earthly attachments like money, property, fame, and even personal relationships begins to fade. They see all physical things as helpful tools, but things that will eventually fall away and be lost.

- Their inner sense of well-being and security has nothing to do with the amount of money or property they currently have. They don't see anything inherently wrong with money and possessions, but they don't allow them to control their sense of well-being and meaning.

> *People suffer at the thought of being without parents,*
> *Without food, or without worth.*
> *Yet this is the very way that*
> *Kings and lords once described themselves.*
> *For one gains by losing,*
> *And loses by gaining.*
> - Lao Tzu

- They use their time, talents, energy and money to serve their callings – those ways they feel called to make a difference. They see everything they give as an offering of gratitude to God.

> *Whatever you do, make it an offering to me – the food you eat, the sacrifices you make,*
> *the help you give, even your suffering.*
> – Bhagavad Gita

- They love others deeply and feel deeply for the death and temporary loss of physical connection with a loved one, but they know the connection is not lost at a spiritual level. They themselves will one day, all too soon, make that transition through the death of their physical bodies into ongoing and eternal life in another state.

- They appreciate and support the miracle of their physical bodies, treating them as a sacred trust and a temple of the divine soul.

- They are not afraid of death. They are not even attached to their own bodies, knowing that they too, like all their physical possessions, will someday pass out of their grasps, and that is just as it should be, because what is still to come is even better, even though they don't really know what it is or even have a need to know. They know that whatever it is, they will still be the one who experiences it and they will still be able to be an expression of love and service.

> *If you realize that all things change,*
> *There is nothing you will try to hold on to.*
> *If you are not afraid of dying,*
> *There is nothing you can't achieve.*
> - LAO TZU

> *Death be not proud, though some have called thee*
> *Mighty and dreadful, for thou art not so,*
> *For, those, whom thou think'st thou dost overthrow,*
> *Die not, poor death, nor yet can'st thou kill me.*
> – JOHN DONNE

- They see that all things are really spiritual and that all experience is for their spiritual evolution.

- They feel intimately connected with a higher power and have a strong sense of being loved, supported by, and guided by that higher power, which is both within them and all around them.

> *You who think to offer your intelligence to God, reconsider.*
> – RUMI

- They feel a sense of immense gratitude and a desire to fearlessly serve others who have not yet awakened to this spiritual reality. However, their service is not rendered with the intent of forcing others to see things their way, or judging them for not seeing things the same way. It is a pure and patient love and compassion that goes about lifting burdens, reassuring troubled minds, and reminding others of their own pure divinity within.

- They don't have any timetables for how long it should take someone to become awakened to this spiritual reality, and they don't have any lines that others can cross that place them too far gone to be loved. They see that everyone is on their own personal journey of human being-ness, and that it is not up to them to decide what another's journey should look like or how long it should take. They see that "It's not over till it's over… and it's never over."

Thoughts on a Station Platform

It ought to be plain
How little you gain
By getting excited
And vexed.
You'll always be late
For the previous train,
And always on time
For the next
- PIET HEIN

Fate laughs saying: "oh really…"
At all our thoughts for the future
As if we're talking child's play and pretend
When speaking of what we shall one day 'become'
For Fate knows that once we meet the Beloved we'll rise in-love so fast,
It'll leave skid marks on our heart's nicely planted patch of plans
Causing us to re-arrange everything we thought we once wanted.
- DREAMING BEAR, BARAKA KANAAN

- They see that people are never done "turning out," but are constantly evolving, even if it appears that they may be losing ground for now.

- They are seen by others as saintly, pure of heart, kind, and compassionate. They dispense few words of advice (especially unsolicited advice), preferring to teach by example. When they do use words, their words are reassuring and affirming of the divinity and power within the other.

- They know that God is impossible to understand in words, but they have a direct personal knowing of God on many levels. In the third person, God is an outside power and ruler, the keeper of order in the universe and the creative power behind all the beauty and diversity of our cosmos. In the second person, God is a friend, coach, or heavenly parent they can pray to and commune with, and with whom they can have a personal relationship. In the first person, God is within them, a

DISTINCTION
Turning Out vs. Evolving

DISTINCTION
God in 3rd, 2nd and 1st Person

seed that is destined to become like that from which it came, the eternal awareness of *I am* that is without beginning of days or end of years.

I have a thousand brilliant lies
For the question:
What is God?
If you think that the Truth can be known from words,
If you think that the Sun and the Ocean
Can pass through that tiny opening called the mouth.
Oh someone should start laughing!
Someone should start wildly laughing–
Now!
- HAFIZ

Last night,
So many tears took flight because of Joy
That the sky got crowded and complained
When I discovered God hiding again in my heart
And I could not cease to celebrate.
– HAFIZ

THE REACTIONS AND BELIEFS OF PEOPLE WITH A BLOCKED OR WEAK SEVENTH CHAKRA

People with a blocked and weak or compromised Seventh Chakra cannot yet see through many illusions related to earthly attachments and separation. As a result they will tend to react in certain ways and believe certain things to be real and those reactions and beliefs will have an impact on their physical bodies and the way they experience life. If you notice any of these reactions or beliefs to be familiar, see it as an opportunity to challenge what you may currently believe to be real. Know that as you commit to a process of daily chakra cleaning and strengthening that you will naturally begin to move away from old beliefs and reactions outlined below and towards those qualities and realizations outlined above. Some of the reactions and beliefs of people with a blocked or weak Seventh Chakra are:

- They are often unable to acknowledge the spiritual aspect of life.

- They find it very difficult to see any purpose in life beyond enjoying what you can and enduring or fighting against the rest.

- They often feel a sense of abandonment by any higher power and anger for all the injustices they see. These become proof that there is no God – or if there is, we're pretty much on our own down here.

- They tend to have an *everyone-for-themselves* attitude.

- Even if they grew up with religious teachings or still have a belief in God and the spiritual, they often feel unworthy and disconnected from the divine.

- They see God as some power outside themselves that rewards or punishes them according to their worthiness.

- They see their worthiness as something they have to constantly struggle to earn and fear that they have unearned it through their thoughts, words, or actions.

- Another way a weak Seventh Chakra can show up is as a form of self-righteousness that places people in separate, distinct groups: those who see things like they do (the *in group*) and those who don't (the unenlightened or unwashed).

- They have a strong attachment to earthly possessions and relationships. Their sense of well-being is highly attached to their level of property and physical security, and to the quality and quantity of their personal relationships. To the extent that they have great possessions and relationships, they live in fear of losing them. To the extent that they do not have great possessions and relationships, they live with a strong belief that this lack is the reason they are not happy and fulfilled. They believe they will be happy and fulfilled once they finally acquire the possessions and relationships they currently lack.

The soul that is attached to anything, however much good there may be in it, will not arrive at the liberty of divine union. For whether it be a strong wire rope or a slender and delicate thread that holds the bird, it matters not, if it really holds it fast; for, until the cord be broken, the bird cannot fly.
— SAINT JOHN OF THE CROSS

SEVENTH CHAKRA QUICK LIST

This is a quick summary of some of the realizations associated with an open and strong Seventh Chakra:

- I am not separate. I am connected to everyone and everything in ways I both understand and don't understand yet.

- I see myself in all others and all others in myself. Everyone and everything can be my teacher, if I am willing and humble enough to be the student.

- Unconditional love and compassion for myself and all others is the only way of being that makes any sense, and if I'm not feeling that, it only means I'm currently seeing and believing an illusion.

- Everything I have been given, my time, my talents, my energy, my earthly possessions, are to be used to serve others in the ways that my soul calls me to do. I can't take any of it with me through the transition of physical death, so I might as well use them to serve my soul's mission.

- I lift burdens, reassure troubled minds, and help others to see through illusions into their own divinity. That's what I do because that's what comes natural. No matter what I may happen to do to make a living, that's what I do to live.

- I am not afraid of death, either mine or others'. I know that I and all others are eternal and eternally connected. Death is just another illusion to see through.

- I can sorrow for the death of a loved one without suffering. The same is true about the loss of property or relationships. I see that sorrow is only evidence that I truly love whereas suffering is what happens when I believe an illusion that things should be different than they are or I should understand why things happen the way they happen.

- It's never my job to decide the path another should take or how their own growth and evolution should best happen.

- I see and experience God on a third person, second person and first person level. I see God everywhere I look- especially when I look into the eyes of another or into the mirror.

When the heart grieves over what it has lost, the spirit rejoices over what it has found.
— SUFI PROVERB

As long as there is something we want to get out of life before we go – a little more money, a little more pleasure, a chance to get in a parting dig at someone we think has hurt us – there will be a terrible struggle with death when it comes. As long as we think we are the body, we will fight to hold onto the body when death comes to wrench it away. The tragedy, of course, is that death is going to take it anyway. So the great teachers in all religions tell us, "Give up your selfish attachments now and be free." Then, when death does come, we can give him what is his without a shadow of regret, and keep for ourselves what is ours, which is love of the Lord.
- EKNATH EASWAREN

(margin) **DISTINCTION** Sorrow vs. Suffering

PART 4:
The Spiral Up Yoga System

21

TOOLS TO STRENGTHEN YOUR CHAKRAS

· ·

The Spiral Up Yoga system has one simple structure:

Do something today, no matter how small, to open and strengthen today's chakra.

You can choose to do just one small thing that may take only a minute or two, or you may want to spend a little longer and add some more power to today's chakra work. You may want to do a few minutes first thing in the morning and a few minutes at night while watching TV or before going to bed. My personal practice usually consists of a few minutes in the morning, either before or after other forms of exercise I do, and then a few more minutes at night. I almost never watch TV from the couch anymore. Instead, if I'm watching TV, I'm sitting or kneeling on the floor doing some of my chakra-strengthening work. If a day comes to a close and I haven't done anything by the time I'm getting ready for bed (which is rare, but it still happens occasionally), I will just do a few minutes before bed. I usually like to do a few minutes before bed every day anyway, because it puts me in a relaxed and peaceful state for a restful and restorative sleep.

The chakra strengthening and cleansing tools I introduce in this chapter are a key element of the Spiral Up Yoga system. These are the different pieces you can pick and choose from on any given day to create your own custom practice. You might think of them as the paints you choose from to paint a picture. So here are the tools, divided into two categories:

1. Those you can do with nothing but your body; nothing additional is needed.

2. Those that require the use of additional tools.

NOTHING REQUIRED BUT YOU

- **Asanas**: Asana is the yoga term for a physical body exercise. This is what most people think of when they think of yoga. The Spiral Up Yoga system organizes the asanas by which chakra they primarily work on. Many asanas will work on more than one chakra, but there is usually a primary chakra being worked on.

- **Toning Sounds**: Specific sounds you make with your own voice. Sound is a vibration, and specific sounds vibrate at frequencies that resonate with the frequencies of specific chakras.

- **Breath Work**: Specific ways of taking conscious control of your breath that are designed to stimulate and strengthen specific chakras. Some breath work can be done while doing asanas, and some can be done alone while you sit at your desk or stand in a line.

- **Emotional Vibration**: This involves consciously choosing to generate a specific quality of emotion by focusing your attention on thoughts that create those emotions. This can be done any time you bring your attention to it. You can do it while driving to work or running errands. You can make that day's emotion your theme for the day and look for ways to focus on and express that emotion during the day. Emotions are feedback on the quality of thoughts we're believing. We are not always aware of what thoughts we're believing, but we're always quite aware of what we're feeling. Consciously focusing your attention on certain thoughts will always create a corresponding emotion. Emotion is basically energy in motion (e-motion), but energy that has a specific message embedded in it, kind of like a radio wave that contains musical content. The chakras are highly impacted by emotional energy.

ANALOGY
Emotions : Radio Waves

- **Mantras**: Mantras are short phrases of one or more words that contain powerful meaning. These words or phrases are spoken silently in your head. This requires your attention to maintain the repetition. Even just a minute or two of focusing your attention on repeating the mantra can have a powerful calming effect on your mind. It can also permeate your energy body with the vibration of the mantra and the meaning contained within the mantra. I will teach you some of my favorite mantras for each chakra, but you can just as easily come up with your own that resonate with the energy of that chakra. Mantras are similar to, but distinct from, emotional vibration methods. The main distinction is that emotional vibration methods are active, while mantras are more passive. Both are useful. The silent repetition of the mantra sustained over a few minutes creates a form of meditative state in the brain. It's like putting the brain in receptive programming mode.

When tormented by painful thoughts, many of us have cried out, "If only I could stop thinking!" But we don't know how. The mind has gotten stuck, and we feel helpless to stop it. All the mind can do is repeat the same thought over and over. Here again, our greatest ally is the mantram. Whenever a destructive thought comes up, repeat the mantram. When the mantram takes hold, the connection between the thought and your attention is broken. A compulsive thought, whether it is anger or depression or a powerful sense-craving, does not really have any power of its own. All the power is in the attention we give – and when we can withdraw our attention, the thought or desire will be helpless to compel us into action.
—EKNATH EASWAREN

- Activities: There are simple little activities that you can do that serve to strengthen your chakras. The suggested activities for each chakra are things that you might ordinarily do in your day anyway, but now they are done with more mindfulness to the impact on your chakras. I'll share with you some of my favorite activities, but once again, use them as options to experiment with. Find those that work well for you, or come up with your own. Some are as easy as taking a warm bath or playing with children.

ADDITIONAL TOOLS REQUIRED

Although these do require a one-time purchase of some additional tools, they are some of the easiest and most direct ways of opening and strengthening the chakras. I do highly recommend you invest in these tools. Information for purchasing them can be found at www.spiralupyoga.com.

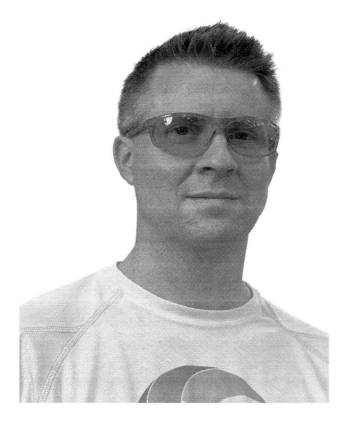

- **Color Glasses**: You can purchase a set of chakra color glasses. These are specially designed colored glasses attuned to the color frequencies of the chakras. All you do is put on that day's color glasses for a minute or two to stimulate the corresponding chakra.

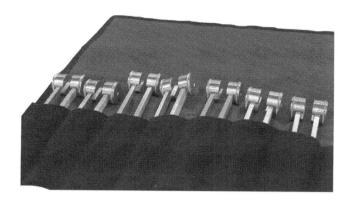

- **Tuning Fork Vibration**: You can purchase a set of tuning forks calibrated specifically to the frequencies of the seven chakras. These can be used by striking the tuning fork, placing it near your ear, and letting the sound vibration permeate your consciousness. I also like to audibly hum the note as I'm listening to it, or combine this with the toning sound (see above), toned audibly at the same frequency as the tuning fork. You can also place the tuning fork stem directly on the bone of the skull behind the ear and have the sound vibration be transmitted directly through the bone instead of through the air. I like to do this once on each side so that I am directly stimulating both hemispheres of my brain. Another way I like to use the tuning forks is to strike them and then place the stem on the appropriate chakra point on my body, letting the vibration permeate directly into my body as it resonates with the frequency of the chakra.

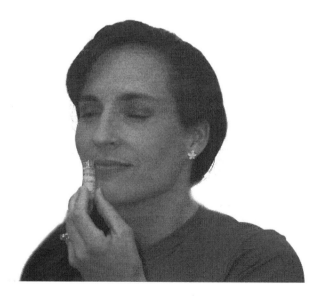

- **Aromatherapy Oils**: Aromatherapy has a long history as a powerful healing modality. You can purchase special oils that have been specifically formulated to stimulate each chakra. All you do is take the appropriate vial of oil for the day,

123

open the lid, and deeply inhale the aroma, which is always a pleasant aroma. Our olfactory nerves are the most direct connection to our deep brains and our memories. There is a lot of research on the powerful impact that smell has on human behavior because it operates on our subconscious minds, triggering memories and mindsets and motivating behavior. I love my aromatherapy set, and this is probably the one tool I use the most often. This one literally takes only a few seconds. It's pleasant to do and very powerful.

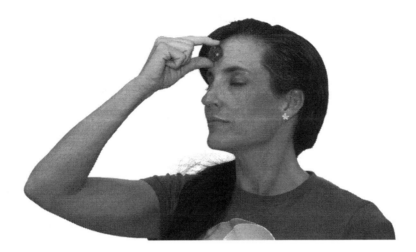

- **Gemstones**: There are specific gemstones that hold frequencies that resonate with the chakras. The use of gemstones in healing has a long history and is seen in many ancient and indigenous cultures, including Egyptian, Chinese, Hawaiian, and Native American cultures. The gemstones, as minerals, are very stable storages of energy frequencies. They can be used almost like recalibration tools to assist the chakras, which are fluid and easily get out of tune, to resonate with the stable frequency of the gemstone. All you need to do is hold the gemstone in your hand and place it on your body near the corresponding chakra. Many energy-healing modalities utilize gemstones in their work. While this may sound a little weird to the logical mind, the use of gemstones is quite scientifically proven. For example, quartz (a gemstone) is routinely used in high-tech equipment, including radio transmitters and receivers, computers, and watches. Its extremely precise and highly stable frequency provides the standard to which the electronic equipment retains its calibration.

WHERE ATTENTION GOES, ENERGY FLOWS

There is an old saying in many of the martial arts and yoga traditions that says, "Where attention goes, energy flows." This is a very important principle when it comes to the link between your spirit body, your energy body, and your physical body. Attention is the focusing of conscious awareness (or spirit) in a particular direction or on a particular person or object. Your attention, which is an aspect of your spirit body, can be focused on any part of your energy or physical body, including your chakras. This will cause the prana energy within and around you to flow more abundantly there. Prana is an intelligent but neutral, receptive form of energy that responds to the active stimulus of your attention.

EXPERIMENT: DIRECTING THE FLOW OF PRANA

Close your eyes and focus your full attention on the palms of your hands. Visualize a ball of energy collecting and forming in your palms. You should begin to feel tingling sensations and maybe warmth. Now direct all your attention to your nose until you feel the same tingling energy sensation there. Now pick another part of your body and direct all your attention there. You might also notice you can feel your pulse in the area you are directing your attention to. With a little patience and practice, you will get more sensitized to the feel of energy in your body and your ability to direct it with your attention.

You don't even need to be limited to directing the flow of prana energy to your own body. Because prana energy is everywhere, flowing through every living thing and interconnecting all, and because you can direct your attention anywhere you choose, you can influence the flow of energy in another person or animal or plant. This is the underlying principle of all energy-healing and distance-healing practices.

EXPERIMENT: TELEPATHIC INFLUENCE

Another fun experiment you might play around with is focusing your attention on a specific person you have a relationship with, perhaps a friend you'd like to have a conversation with or someone you'd like to return your call or e-mail. Send the person loving energy, and imagine her feeling a calm sense of peace wherever she is. Send a specific intention that you would like to have a conversation or a response to your message. Then just wait to see what happens. You might be surprised at how often the person will contact you within the next few hours. Alternatively, you might try calling her. She will often say something like, "Oh, I was just thinking of you and planning to give you a call." This has likely already happened to you on many occasions. Of course you can't override another person's free will, but consciously directing your attention to other people in a loving manner will influence them. The more you and the other person are in your receptive flow state of mind, as opposed to a hard-pressing, analytical churn mode, the more quickly and clearly these telepathic connections can be sensed.

The point of these experiments is to provide you with a personal experience of consciously directing energy so that it moves beyond just a theory or an intellectual understanding and becomes something you realize directly.

THE POWER KICKER TO ANY OF THE SPIRAL UP YOGA TOOLS

Regardless of the tools that you choose to use on any given day, the more you are able to consciously direct your attention during the exercise to the relevant chakra, the more powerful the exercise will become. The exercises will still impact your chakra even if your attention is scattered, so don't worry that you're wasting your time if you don't have full control of your attention during the exercises. Think of your conscious focus of attention on your chakra as a power kicker to your work. So, for example, if today is Second Chakra day, and I'm doing a toning exercise, I would want to close my eyes as I voice the sound and direct my attention to the location of my Second Chakra (the lower abdomen, about two inches below the navel and at the depth of my spine) to the point where I could feel that area vibrating and tingling. I would want to visualize my Second Chakra as a swirling ball of bright orange energy becoming brighter as I do the exercise. I may also imagine that little dark specks of impurity that have collected there are broken up and cast off, restoring the chakra to a clearer, purer and brighter state. These aren't just simple visualizations, they are intentions that activate and direct prana to respond as you're directing it to.

㉓

THE SPIRAL UP YOGA WEEKLY CYCLE

- -

Warning: If you're the impatient type who just wants to get to the specific how-to stuff so you can try it out, and have skipped to this section of the book without reading all that came before this, I want to warn you that you will not get as much out of doing the practice without first becoming familiar with all the content I've presented up to this point. If you want to proceed without that foundation, go ahead; this is a book, not a class where I can control the order of things. But even if you do start playing around with the actual practice of Spiral Up Yoga, I highly encourage you to go back and get familiar with the content I've presented because it will allow you to get much more out of your practice.

Now, let's jump in and start creating your own customized Spiral Up Yoga practice. Next I'll go through each of the seven days of the week and give you tools you can choose from to create your own practice. The point is not to try to use all of the tools every day, but to pick a few and do them with as much of your conscious attention as you can.

Remember, there is only one simple structure to this system:

Do something, however small, to open and strengthen today's chakra.

That's it. What you actually do on any given day will be totally up to you. Experiment with the various tools, and you'll begin to find your favorites (for now). Change it up as you want to so that it never becomes boring and your practice evolves with you.

If you miss a day (or even a few days), don't worry, and don't give up. Just pick up where you are. If it's Wednesday, it's Third Chakra day, so just use a Third Chakra tool of your choosing. You don't have to start back at First Chakra and make up for the missed days. Please don't turn this into yet another stick to beat yourself up with if you miss a day or even a week. You don't need any new ways of shaming yourself. In fact, you don't even need your old ways of shaming yourself!

WHAT WAS I LEARNING?

Speaking of shaming yourself, I'll share a little trick that I find very helpful when I find myself in a mode of self-shame over past actions. Instead of asking, "What was I thinking?" I ask, "What was I learning (even if I wasn't aware of it at the time)?" Life is a learn-by-actual-experience school in which there are no mistakes, only lessons learned and relearned (and relearned). When a toddler is learning to walk, falling a lot is a joyful part of

ANALOGY
Learning to Walk: Learning to Love

ite the truth: just like a child learns to walk by falling, we are here on earth learning to
love as God loves. That requires that we get an unlimited number of chances to practice
loving in all sorts of situations. So stop shaming yourself for your past mistakes. If you
need permission to stop it, I hereby give you permission. Better yet, authorize yourself –
you don't need anyone else's permission or authority.

State after me: "I hereby authorize myself to stop shaming myself, and instead look for how
this situation can teach me how to love more." Like any new routine you try to introduce, it
takes some time before it becomes second nature, so don't mentally bully yourself if your
practice isn't perfectly consistent. Any work you do to consciously open and strengthen
your chakras is beneficial to you on all levels – body, mind, and soul. And any work you do
now is more than you were doing before, so it's all good!

The weekly cycle is really simple:

- Monday is First Chakra day

- Tuesday is Second Chakra day

- Wednesday is Third Chakra day

- Thursday is Fourth Chakra day

- Friday is Fifth Chakra day

- Saturday is Sixth Chakra day

- Sunday is Seventh Chakra day

Next we'll go day by day through all seven days, detailing all of the tools at your disposal
for custom building your own personal practice.

24

MONDAY: FIRST CHAKRA DAY

FIRST CHAKRA OVERVIEW

The First Chakra deals with your physical survival and safety, so strengthening the First Chakra is all about feeling safe, secure, supported, and grounded. Think of your First Chakra as your root system that connects you to the unlimited support of the earth and supports you in all your activities and pursuits. The First Chakra deserves some extra care and attention because without sufficient energy in the First Chakra, all the other chakras suffer. The First Chakra acts as a pump at the base of the chakra system that helps energy rise along the spine and to the crown of the head. If this base pump is weak, work done on the other chakras won't be as effective.

THEME FOR MONDAYS: TRUE SECURITY WITHIN

Begin all Mondays with this theme (or choose another phrase from the mantras below, or use your own phrase that fits with the subject matter of the chakra). Make today about noticing all the ways your true security comes from within, and all the ways you may lose track of that as you seek security in other people, places, or pursuits. Let this theme permeate your thinking both while doing specific Spiral Up Yoga practices and throughout the rest of your activities today. With this as your theme, you'll likely be surprised at how many ways you begin to notice this and how many things and people become your teachers of this principle of the First Chakra. When the student is ready, the teacher appears. Notice how true this is for you as everything around you becomes a teacher of true security coming from within and you become the student, really seeing this on many new levels.

> *To be truly secure, we must begin to find a source of security within ourselves. Even the bravest among us have many fears. Behind the attachment to money or possessions, for example, you will always find the fear of loss. Attachment to prestige brings the nagging fear of what others think of us. The thirst for power feeds the fear that others may be stronger. Every self-centered desire brings the fear that we may not get what we desire. One could make a Sears catalog of these fears, but all stem from one fatal superstition: thinking of ourselves as merely physical creatures, separate from the rest of life. As our sense of oneness with the rest of life deepens, we step out of the world of fear to live in the world of love.*
> - EKNATH EASWAREN

EMOTIONAL VIBRATION

Focus your thoughts on being safe, secure, and supported by life and by others; on being grounded, relaxed, and able to handle whatever comes your way, knowing that everything that happens is for your learning and that life is for you, not against you. You can't focus your attention on thoughts without having an emotional response that will allow you to literally feel in your body the vibration of the thoughts you are focusing on.

TONING

Sing or tone the word "grow," holding out the "oh" sound as long as your breath allows. The word "grow" both gives the right vowel sound to tone and has meaning related to the First Chakra. Just like a plant can't grow until it is planted and rooted, you can't really grow unless you are grounded, rooted, supported, and you know that you're ultimately safe and secure, even if you don't always feel that way because you're believing insecure thoughts (as we all do at times). As you hold out the "oh" sound, bring your attention to your First Chakra and try to feel it vibrating and glowing. Imagine the red glow getting brighter and stronger.

BREATH

Monday's breath is called the "mudra lock." Here's how you do it:

> Sit, kneel, or stand. Inhale deeply into the lower abdomen. Now, hold the breath in and tightly squeeze everything from navel to anus. Hold this squeeze for a few counts. Exhale, and with the breath held out, repeat the squeezing and holding for a few more counts. Inhale and relax. Repeat as desired.

> The mudra lock breath helps to stimulate the First Chakra, which acts like an energy pump for all the higher chakras. The squeezing and holding with the breath held in and out literally pumps energy from the base of your spine all the way to the crown of your head. Pay attention to the feel of the energy in your body as you do this. See if you can feel it move up your spine and to the top of your head. Imagine it's like one of those carnival games where you hit the base with a hammer and see how high you can make the ball go.

> You can do this breath any time during the day: at your desk, in your car, or even in the shower.

MANTRA

Here are a few that you could use, or come up with your own that relate to the overall theme of the First Chakra. (To understand the best way to use the mantra, see the discussion of mantras in the "Tools to Strengthen Your Chakras" chapter).

"All is well."

"True safety within."

"True security within."

"Relax; it's all good."

"I am safe no matter what."

"Nothing truly mine can ever be taken away."

"Anything that can be taken away is not truly mine."

ACTIVITIES

- Reconnect your body to the earth in some direct physical way. Walk barefoot in your back yard or a nearby park, sit against the trunk of a tree and connect with the energy of the earth, or spend time outdoors and in nature, noticing all the ways that you are like nature.

- Reflect on the question: "What is truly mine?" with your definition being, "Anything that can never be taken from me." Write down your insights.

COLOR GLASSES

If you have purchased a set of chakra color glasses, put on the red glasses and see your world through the lens of red. Feel it stimulating and resonating with your First Chakra.

TUNING FORK VIBRATION

If you have purchased a set of chakra-calibrated tuning forks, strike the First Chakra tuning fork and place it near your ear. Imagine your First Chakra growing a brighter and stronger red. Strike it again and place the stem on your skull behind your right ear and then again on your skull behind your left ear. Let the vibrations stimulate and permeate both hemispheres of your brain. Next, strike it again and place the stem against the bottom of your spine on your lower back. Allow the physical vibration to permeate into the tissues of your body and imagine it stimulating and strengthening your First Chakra and breaking up any crustiness that may have collected or dimmed its light.

AROMATHERAPY

If you have purchased a set of chakra-calibrated aromatherapy oils, open the First Chakra vial and inhale the aroma deeply, letting the aroma permeate your entire being. Imagine it stimulating and strengthening your First Chakra. Try covering your left nostril and inhaling through the right nostril, and then reversing and inhaling through the left nostril.

GEMSTONES

If you have purchased a set of chakra gemstones, grab the First Chakra stone and hold it at the bottom of your spine on your back. Imagine it stimulating and strengthening your First Chakra. Imagine your chakra re-calibrating itself to the highly stable vibration of the gemstone, just as a high quality watch keeps accurate time by constantly re-calibrating to the quartz crystal inside it.

ASANAS

Refer to the separate Asana Guide that follows this section. Choose a few and experiment with them. Add more later as you want to, or mix it up as you wish. You can see videos of these asanas at spiralupyoga.com. This book contains seven asanas per chakra. There are many others that you can add as well. See the website for details.

25

TUESDAY: SECOND CHAKRA DAY

SECOND CHAKRA OVERVIEW

The Second Chakra deals with issues of self-worth, relationships, pleasure, sexuality, and creativity. The Second Chakra supports the reproductive organs, bladder, and kidneys. Strengthening the Second Chakra is all about feeling worthy, valued, and loved by ourselves. Notice I said "ourselves," not "others." We can only love others to the extent we first love ourselves. Seeking the love of others when we don't love ourselves is really neediness, not true love.

THEME FOR TUESDAYS: INNATELY WORTHY

Begin all Tuesdays with this theme (or choose another phrase from the mantras below, or use your own phrase that fits with the subject matter of the chakra). Make today about noticing all the ways your true worth is innate and untouchable, and all the ways you may lose track of that as you seek feelings of worthiness in your accomplishments and your relationships. Let this theme permeate your thinking both while doing specific Spiral Up Yoga practices and throughout the rest of your activities today. With this as your theme, you'll likely be surprised at how many ways you begin to notice this and how many things and people become your teachers of this principle of the Second Chakra. When the student is ready, the teacher appears. Notice how true this is for you as everything around you becomes a teacher of true innate worthiness and you become the student, really seeing this on many new levels.

Accepting yourself as you are doesn't mean inaction, it means not wasting time justifying how you got to where you are now. What we resist, persists. The more you hate something, the more bound you are to it. The more you love something, the more free you are.
– Eknath Easwaren

EMOTIONAL VIBRATION

Focus your thoughts on being innately worthy, regardless of past actions, and being able to qualify yourself to do whatever your soul desires. Forgive yourself for your past mistakes and feel the new energy that comes from laying down that burden of guilt. Feel confident that if there are any actions you need to take to apologize or right a wrong, you will. Instead of, "What was I thinking?" ask, "What was I learning?" Focus on all you have to be grateful for and on the flow and grace of life that is waiting to take you onward and upward from your past. See yourself flowing with life, flowing around obstacles, and not having to know ahead of time everything that is around the next bend. Just be confident that you are open, receptive, worthy, and able to respond appropriately to whatever may come. Now your natural creativity can flow from within you – creativity that was previously trapped behind the jail walls of self-imposed guilt and unworthiness.

TONING

Sing or tone the word "move," holding out the "ooo" sound as long as your breath allows. The word "move" both gives the right vowel sound to tone for the Second Chakra and has meaning related to the Second Chakra. As you release your guilt and illusions of unworthiness, you release the anchors that have kept you from moving onward and upward. You are now free to move with greater freedom in the present moment and not stay stuck in the past. Holding yourself back and withdrawing from expressing your soul doesn't serve anyone. As you hold out the "ooo" sound, bring your attention to your Second Chakra and try to feel it vibrating and glowing. Imagine the orange glow getting brighter and stronger.

BREATH

Tuesday's breath is called the "bellows breath." Here's how you do it:

Lie on your back. Slowly expand your lower abdomen on all four sides like a bellows opening, silently drawing in air through your nose. Hold the breath in for a few counts while fully expanded. Then slowly compress the bellows until all the air is gone. Use your core muscles to push out every last bit of air you can and hold the air out for a few counts before repeating. This is meant to be long, deep, slow breathing. You can also place your hands above your Second Chakra and make that the center of the rise and fall of your bellows. This breath can also be done standing or sitting.

The goal here is to focus your attention on moving your diaphragm and expanding your lower abdominal cavity rather than on breathing in air through your nose or mouth. The air is just silently drawn in due to the vacuum that has been created by opening the bellows and silently pressed out as the bellows is slowly closed.

You can do this breath any time during the day: at your desk, sitting in your car, or lying in your bed or the floor.

MANTRA

Here are a few that you could use, or come up with your own that relate to the overall theme of the Second Chakra. (To understand the best way to use the mantra, see the discussion of mantras in the "Tools to Strengthen Your Chakras" chapter).

"Innately worthy."

"Nothing to forgive."

"Onward, upward."

"Flow with life."

"Self-love."

ACTIVITIES

- Take a relaxing bath.

- Play music that relaxes and inspires you.

- Listen to the sound of ocean waves for a few minutes while you flow back and forth, becoming the ocean. (You can find audio clips online for free.)

- Take a relaxing stroll in the moonlight by yourself or with a loved one.

COLOR GLASSES

If you have purchased a set of chakra color glasses, put on the orange glasses and see your world through the lens of orange. Feel it stimulating and resonating with your Second Chakra.

TUNING FORK VIBRATION

If you have purchased a set of chakra-calibrated tuning forks, strike the Second Chakra tuning fork and place it near your ear. Imagine your Second Chakra glowing a brighter and stronger orange. Strike it again and place the stem on your skull behind your right ear and then again on your skull behind your left ear. Let the vibrations stimulate and permeate both hemispheres of your brain. Next, strike it again and place the stem against your lower abdomen, about two inches directly below your navel. Allow the physical vibration to permeate into the tissues of your body and imagine it opening and strengthening your Second Chakra.

AROMATHERAPY

If you have purchased a set of chakra-calibrated aromatherapy oils, open the Second Chakra vial and inhale the aroma deeply, letting the aroma permeate your entire being. Imagine it stimulating and strengthening your Second Chakra. Try covering your left nostril and inhaling through the right nostril and then reversing and inhaling through the left nostril.

GEMSTONES

If you have purchased a set of chakra gemstones, grab the Second Chakra stone and hold it to your Second Chakra point, about two inches directly below your navel. Imagine it stimulating and strengthening your Second Chakra. Imagine your chakra re-calibrating itself to the highly stable vibration of the gemstone, just as a high quality watch keeps accurate time by constantly re-calibrating to the quartz crystal inside it.

ASANAS

Refer to the separate Asana Guide that follows this section. Choose a few and experiment with them. Add more later as you want to, or mix it up as you wish. You can see videos of these asanas at spiralupyoga.com. This book contains seven asanas per chakra. There are many others that you can add as well. See the website for details.

WEDNESDAY: THIRD CHAKRA DAY

. . . .

THIRD CHAKRA OVERVIEW

The Third Chakra deals with issues of willpower, ambition, and action. Strengthening the Third Chakra is all about feeling empowered and confident to take desired action in your world. The Third Chakra supports the stomach, liver, gall bladder, and pancreas. It is located in the solar plexus, about two inches above your navel. This is the seat of the physical self and at the junction between the voluntary and involuntary nervous system. It is also connected through the major vagus nerve to the neocortex, which makes it sensitive to stress. If the stress is prolonged, deterioration of the internal organs supported by the Third Chakra will typically occur. The Third Chakra also controls the body's appetite and metabolism functions, so it is highly likely that if your physical body has metabolism issues and your weight is very far off the range of normal for your body type (in either direction), your Third Chakra has become weakened or blocked.

As a side note, if you're not yet aware of which of the three body types you are, it would help to know that so you are using the right standard for your current physical body condition. There are three body types:

1. Ectomorph: small-sized frame, bones, and body mass

2. Mesomorph: middle-sized frame, bones, and body mass

3. Endomorph: large-sized frame, bones, and body mass

All three body types exist on a spectrum of balanced and healthy to unbalanced and unhealthy. Don't try to compare yourself to another body type, or you will just frustrate yourself by trying to reach a standard for which your physical body is not designed. That would be like a rose trying to become a lilac. To learn more about body types, just do an Internet search for "the three body types."

THEME FOR WEDNESDAYS: SERVICE IN ACTION

Begin all Wednesdays with this theme (or choose another phrase from the mantras below, or use your own phrase that fits with the subject matter of the chakra). Make today about noticing all the ways you are already in action serving others and other ways you can more powerfully be in action serving others. See how you don't need anyone else's permission to be in action serving. Let this theme permeate your thinking both while doing specific Spiral Up Yoga practices and throughout the rest of your activities today. With this as your theme, you'll likely be surprised at how many ways you begin to notice this and how many things and people become your teachers of this principle of the Third Chakra. When the student is ready, the teacher appears. Notice how true this is for you as everything around you becomes a teacher of service in action and you become the student, really seeing this on many new levels.

It is not so much work that tires us, but ego-driven work. When we are selfishly involved, we cannot help worrying, we cannot help getting overly concerned about our success or failure. The preoccupation with results makes us tense, and our anxiety exhausts us.

The Gita is essentially a call to action. But it is a call to selfless action, that is, action without any selfish attachments to the results. It asks us to do our best, yet never allow ourselves to become involved in whether things work out the way we want.

It takes practice to learn this skill, but once you have it, as Gandhi says, you will never lose your nerve. The sense of inadequacy goes, and the question "Am I equal to this job?" will not arise. It is enough that the job needs to be done and that you are doing your best to get it done.
– EKNATH EASWAREN

EMOTIONAL VIBRATION

Focus your thoughts on being innately powerful and capable of making a positive difference for others. See yourself being fearless about bringing out what is authentically you. See yourself as confident and accomplished, radiating power in the service of others. As you do, bring your attention to your Third Chakra and imagine a bright internal sun shining forth with warmth and light.

TONING

Sing or tone the word "God," holding out the "ah" sound as long as your breath allows. The word "God" both gives the right vowel sound to tone for the Third Chakra and has meaning related to the Third Chakra. As you release your self-conscious focus and instead focus on how you can authentically serve others with power, you open yourself up for being a more powerful instrument that God can use to bless the lives of others. As you hold out the "ah" sound, bring your attention to your Third Chakra and try to feel it vibrating and glowing. Imagine the yellow glow getting brighter and stronger.

BREATH

Wednesday's breath is called the "breath of fire." Here's how you do it:

Any position is fine: standing, sitting, kneeling, or lying on your back. The breath of fire is a rapid, steady, but deep inhale and exhale through the nose into the Third Chakra area (the solar plexus). Try to do about two inhales and two exhales per second. Keep it up for a minute or two. In/Out, In/Out, In/Out, In/Out as your abdomen is pumping in and out. The breath of fire is a highly energizing breath that gets your energy stimulated and flowing. Think of it as stoking the fire in your belly (your solar plexus), which is your internal sun and power generator.

You can do this breath any time during the day: at your desk, sitting in your car, or lying in your bed. The breath of fire is also a common breath used during some of the asanas.

MANTRA

Here are a few that you could use, or come up with your own that relate to the overall theme of the Third Chakra. (To understand the best way to use the mantra, see the discussion of mantras in the "Tools to Strengthen Your Chakras" chapter).

"Service in action."

"Inner sun."

"Inner power."

"Why not me?"

"Fearless."

"Nothing to fear."

ACTIVITIES

- Sun gazing: Spend a few minutes gazing directly but softly at the rising or setting sun without any sunglasses. The UV rays during the first hour of sunrise and last hour of sunset are harmless to your eyes (and skin). In fact, the spectrum of solar radiation during the first and last hour of sunlight is very beneficial to all three of your bodies (physical, energy, and spirit). Visualize the warm energy of the sun entering through your eyes and skin and collecting in your solar plexus.

This is actually an ancient practice practiced by cultures including Mayan, Egyptian and Indian. All living things on the earth get their energy for life from the sun, either directly or indirectly. Our food is really sun energy that has been converted into food energy, and then when we eat it is re-converted into body energy. But we, like plants, are designed to be able to take in sun energy directly without having to use food as an intermediary. There are people alive today who have taken this principle very far to the point of living healthily for many years without any food, just getting their energy directly from the sun through sun gazing. There is one man from India who has made himself a test case to be studied by NASA about living directly off of sun energy. NASA is interested because this has important implications for long-term space travel where food supply becomes a limitation.

- Do something physical that focuses on your body, perhaps some form of exercise (like yoga).

- If you enjoy gardening, it is a great Third Chakra strengthener to spend time outdoors and see your proper role as a gardener partnering with God to bring about a fruitful harvest. You realize that you're only doing about one percent of the total work required to grow a crop or flowers, but that your one percent is crucial to the outcome. The same is true with anything else you want to create in your life. (I wrote an entire twelve-unit e-course built around this understanding and getting clear on what our one-percent role in creating our lives consists of. If you would like to explore that, you can learn more at www.sunflowerexperiment.com).

COLOR GLASSES

If you have purchased a set of chakra color glasses, put on the yellow glasses and see your world through the lens of yellow. Feel it stimulating and resonating with your Third Chakra.

TUNING FORK VIBRATION

If you have purchased a set of chakra-calibrated tuning forks, strike the Third Chakra tuning fork and place it near your ear. Hum along to the tone, trying to feel the vibration in the Third Chakra. Imagine your Third Chakra glowing a brighter and stronger yellow. Strike it again and place the stem on your skull behind your right ear and then again on your skull behind your left ear. Let the vibrations stimulate and permeate both hemispheres of your brain. Next, strike it again and place the stem against your solar plexus, about two inches directly above your navel. Allow the physical vibration to permeate into the tissues of your body and imagine it stimulating and strengthening your Third Chakra.

AROMATHERAPY

If you have purchased a set of chakra-calibrated aromatherapy oils, open the Third Chakra vial and inhale the aroma deeply, letting the aroma permeate your entire being. Imagine it stimulating and strengthening your Third Chakra. Try covering your left nostril and inhaling through the right nostril, and then reversing and inhaling through the left nostril.

GEMSTONES

If you have purchased a set of chakra gemstones, grab the Third Chakra stone and hold it to your Third Chakra point, about two inches directly above your navel. Imagine it stimulating and strengthening your Third Chakra. Imagine your chakra re-calibrating itself to the highly stable vibration of the gemstone, just as a high quality watch keeps accurate time by constantly re-calibrating to the quartz crystal inside it.

ASANAS

Refer to the separate Asana Guide that follows this section. Choose a few and experiment with them. Add more later as you want to, or mix it up as you wish. You can see videos of these asanas at spiralupyoga.com. This book contains seven asanas per chakra. There are many others that you can add as well. See the website for details.

27

THURSDAY: FOURTH CHAKRA DAY

FOURTH CHAKRA OVERVIEW

The Fourth Chakra deals with issues of love, compassion, and connection. The Fourth Chakra lies directly in the middle position of the seven-chakra ladder with three below and three above. The three lower chakras are sometimes called the body chakras, and the three above the mind chakras. The heart chakra is what links body and mind together. It facilitates the balance of emotion with logic and the real with the ideal.

THEME FOR THURSDAYS: LOVING WHAT IS

Begin all Thursdays with this theme (or choose another phrase from the mantras below, or use your own phrase that fits with the subject matter of the chakra). Make today about noticing all the ways you do love what is, and all the ways you are not currently loving what is. How you can begin to love those aspects of your current experience of life more? Notice your tendency to complain, and see how you can turn complaining into gratitude. Let this theme permeate your thinking both while doing specific Spiral Up Yoga practices and throughout the rest of your activities today. With this as your theme, you'll likely be surprised at how many ways you begin to notice ways to love what is and how many things and people become your teachers of this principle of the Fourth Chakra. When the student is ready, the teacher appears. Notice how true this is for you as everything around you becomes a teacher of loving what is, and you become the student, really seeing this on many new levels.

> *Because I know that time is always time*
> *And place is always and only place*
> *And what is actual is actual only for one time*
> *And only for one place*
> *I rejoice that things are as they are.*
> -T.S. ELLIOT

EMOTIONAL VIBRATION

Focus your thoughts on being innately loving and compassionate. If you want to feel love and compassion, how do you go about doing that? What thoughts help you create that feeling? Maybe it's thinking about your children, spouse, or parents. See yourself connected at the heart level to all others and as no better or no worse than any other, just a fellow student of the earth school who is learning how to love more fully. As you do, bring your attention to your Fourth Chakra and imagine a bright and warm green light emanating from your heart area, nurturing all with love, including yourself.

TONING

Sing or tone the word "raise," holding out the "ay" sound as long as your breath allows. The word "raise" both gives the right vowel sound to tone for the Fourth Chakra and has meaning related to the Fourth Chakra. See your love and compassion as raising your own moods and sense of connection, as well as raising other people you interact with to a higher level of love and compassion. All things grow with love. As you hold out the "ay" sound, bring your attention to your Fourth Chakra and try to feel it vibrating and glowing. Imagine the green glow getting brighter and stronger.

BREATH

Thursday's breath is called the "ten-ten-ten" breath. Here's how you do it:

> Any position is fine: standing, sitting, kneeling, or lying on your back. Inhale slowly and deeply for a count of ten. Then hold the breath in for a count of ten, then exhale slowly for a count of ten and repeat as many times as desired. This is a balancing breath that helps to restore a balance of body and mind, as well as a balance of energy in the Fourth Chakra, which is the center, or balancing, chakra.

> You can do this breath any time during the day: at your desk, sitting in your car, or lying in your bed.

MANTRA

Here are a few that you could use, or come up with your own that relate to the overall theme of the Fourth Chakra. (To understand the best way to use the mantra, see the discussion of mantras in the "Tools to Strengthen Your Chakras" chapter).

"Loving what is."

"Love and compassion."

"Raise me up."

"Condemn not."

"Mercy for all."

"Allow, accept, appreciate, act."

ACTIVITIES

- Do something small or large to serve someone else. Make it anonymous if you can, but it's not necessary. See a mess? Clean it up, even though you might see it as someone else's responsibility.

- Find little ways to express your love and appreciation like writing a thank-you card, calling a friend to express your love and appreciation, or telling your spouse or child how much you love and appreciate them just the way they are.

- Turn an annoyance into something for which you feel love and gratitude. For example, a messy home with toys and clothes and dirty dishes that kids have left all over. Instead of getting annoyed, see if you can see deeper and realize that the only reason you have the mess is because you are privileged enough to have children. Then you can turn what was an annoyance into the very reason you have to feel love and gratitude. Maybe you get annoyed by your spouse who squeezes the toothpaste tube from the middle, or puts the toilet paper roll on the dispenser the way you don't like, or leaves dirty clothes on the floor, or whatever little things they do that tend to annoy you. Turn those very things into physical reminders of how blessed you are to have a spouse, without which you wouldn't get to be annoyed by these little things.

COLOR GLASSES

If you have purchased a set of chakra color glasses, put on the green glasses and see your world through the lens of green. Feel it stimulating and resonating with your Fourth Chakra.

TUNING FORK VIBRATION

If you have purchased a set of chakra-calibrated tuning forks, strike the Fourth Chakra tuning fork and place it near your ear. Hum along to the tone, trying to feel the vibration in the Fourth Chakra. Imagine your Fourth Chakra glowing a brighter and stronger green. Strike it again and place the stem on your skull behind your right ear and then again on your skull behind your left ear. Let the vibrations stimulate and permeate both hemispheres of your brain. Next, strike it again and place the stem at the Fourth Chakra point on your chest, right between your breasts at the level of your heart. Allow the physical vibration to permeate into the tissues of your body, and imagine it stimulating and strengthening your Fourth Chakra.

AROMATHERAPY

If you have purchased a set of chakra-calibrated aromatherapy oils, open the Fourth Chakra vial and inhale the aroma deeply, letting the aroma permeate your entire being. Imagine it stimulating and strengthening your Fourth Chakra. Try covering your left nostril and inhaling through the right nostril, and then reversing and inhaling through the left nostril.

GEMSTONES

If you have purchased a set of chakra gemstones, grab the Fourth Chakra stone and hold it to your Fourth Chakra point, between your breasts at heart level. Imagine it stimulating and strengthening your Fourth Chakra. Imagine your chakra re-calibrating itself to the highly stable vibration of the gemstone, just as a high quality watch keeps accurate time by constantly re-calibrating to the quartz crystal inside it.

ASANAS

Refer to the separate Asana Guide that follows this section. Choose a few and experiment with them. Add more later as you want to, or mix it up as you wish. You can see videos of these asanas at spiralupyoga.com. This book contains seven asanas per chakra. There are many others that you can add as well. See the website for details.

FRIDAY: FIFTH CHAKRA DAY

FIFTH CHAKRA OVERVIEW

The Fifth Chakra deals with the power of speaking truth and expressing yourself with your words and actions. The Fifth Chakra, being between the Fourth Chakra (heart) and the Sixth Chakra (mind), reflects how open a person's heart and mind are and how harmoniously a person lives from both heart and mind.

THEME FOR FRIDAYS: EXPRESSING DEEP TRUTH

Begin all Fridays with this theme (or choose another phrase from the mantras below, or use your own phrase that fits with the subject matter of the chakra). Make today about noticing all the ways you are already expressing deep truth in your words and actions, and all the ways you may be restraining yourself and not expressing your deep truth. By deep truth, I mean the truth that lies at a deeper level than surface appearances. Expressing your critical and demeaning thoughts to someone is not expressing deep truth; it is merely expressing your insecure thinking, which is an illusion not grounded in truth at all. Using your words and actions to encourage or reassure yourself or others in an uplifting way is an example of expressing deep truth. Let this theme permeate your thinking both while doing specific Spiral Up Yoga practices and throughout the rest of your activities today. With this as your theme, you'll likely be surprised at how many ways you begin to notice the truth of the theme and how many things and people become your teachers of this principle of the Fifth Chakra. When the student is ready, the teacher appears. Notice how true this is for you as everything around you becomes a teacher of expressing deep truth and you become the student, really seeing this on many new levels.

> *O I could sing such grandeurs and glories about you!*
> *You have not known what you are,*
> *You have slumber'd upon yourself all your life,*
> *Your eyelids have been the same as closed most of the time…*
> *Whoever you are! Claim your own at any hazard!*
> *These shows of the East and West are tame compared to you,*
> *These immense meadows, these interminable rivers,*
> *You are immense and interminable as they…*
> - WALT WHITMAN

EMOTIONAL VIBRATION

Focus your thoughts on seeing, speaking, and facing the truth in all forms – not just surface appearances, but the deep truth, which is this: you and all others are divine beings having a human experience, and we're all here learning how to love. Part of the lesson is learning how to work together even when we're all seeing illusions, both shared and personal. See your Fifth Chakra glowing a bright sky blue as you become a source of clarity and truth to yourself and to others. Imagine, as you begin to face and speak deep truth, that others begin to respond by wanting to assist you in creating what you want, because by so doing, they are assisted in becoming what they deeply want to be.

TONING

Sing or tone the word "thee," holding out the "ee" sound as long as your breath allows. The word "thee" both gives the right vowel sound to tone for the Fifth Chakra and has meaning related to the Fifth Chakra. "Thee" is a form of great respect reserved for royalty and deity. When you tone "thee," you are calling upon the divine being within you to help you see, face, and speak deep truth. You are also seeing others you serve as worthy of your highest respect. As you hold out the "ee" sound, bring your attention to your Fifth Chakra and try to feel it vibrating and glowing. Imagine the sky blue glow getting brighter and stronger.

BREATH

Friday's breath is called the "chin-to-chest" breath. Here's how you do it:

> Any position is fine: standing, sitting, or kneeling. Inhale slowly as you both expand and raise your chest and lower your chin until it touches your chest. It should feel like you are placing physical pressure on your Fifth Chakra. Keep chin held to chest as you hold the breath in for a few counts. Then exhale as you raise your chin and lower your chest. Repeat as desired.

> You can do this breath any time during the day: at your desk, sitting in your car, or while watching TV.

MANTRA

Here are a few that you could use, or come up with your own that relate to the overall theme of the Fifth Chakra. (To understand the best way to use the mantra, see the discussion of mantras in the "Tools to Strengthen Your Chakras" chapter).

"Express deep truth."

"Truth is kind."

"Integrity."

"My words reassure others of their divinity."

ACTIVITIES

- Sing out loud. Sing along to your favorite songs. Sing in the shower or the car. Belt it out.

- Write in a journal or log about anything you want to express. Be honest about what you're feeling, even if it seems petty. Get your thoughts onto paper.

- Start a "Book of Insights" where you write down insights and creative ideas you have so they are captured and put into words.

- Use your words to reassure someone who is currently caught up in stressful thinking due to believing an illusion and forgetting who they really are. Maybe it's you that you need to reassure.

- Write down requests you could make of others to help you create something you want to create. Explore ways in which your request can serve those others, not just you. Now make a request to someone, expressing how it will serve that person and others. Do it in a conversation or an e-mail, but remain unattached to the response you get. Just know that regardless of the response you get, you are strengthening your request-making muscle.

- *Advanced but powerful:* Get a pen and paper and write down "Lies I have been telling/hiding from others" and "Lies I have been telling/hiding from myself" and see what comes up. Then conduct an experiment: have any conversation that you feel you could have that would allow you to cross one of the lies off your list. See what happens. This is not an exercise in how to shame yourself more. Quite the opposite; it is an experiment in realizing how much kinder the truth is than the lie.

COLOR GLASSES

If you have purchased a set of chakra color glasses, put on the blue glasses and see your world through the lens of blue. Feel it stimulating and resonating with your Fifth Chakra.

TUNING FORK VIBRATION

If you have purchased a set of chakra-calibrated tuning forks, strike the Fifth Chakra tuning fork and place it near your ear. Hum along to the tone, trying to feel the vibration in the Fifth Chakra. Imagine your Fifth Chakra glowing a brighter and stronger blue. Strike it again and place the stem on your skull behind your right ear and then again on your skull behind your left ear. Let the vibrations stimulate and permeate both hemispheres of your brain. Next, strike it again and place the stem at the Fifth Chakra point on your neck, about one inch below the chin. Allow the physical vibration to permeate into the tissues of your body, and imagine it stimulating and strengthening your Fifth Chakra.

AROMATHERAPY

If you have purchased a set of chakra-calibrated aromatherapy oils, open the Fifth Chakra vial and inhale the aroma deeply, letting the aroma permeate your entire being. Imagine it stimulating and strengthening your Fifth Chakra. Try covering your left nostril and inhaling through the right nostril, and then reversing and inhaling through the left nostril.

GEMSTONES

If you have purchased a set of chakra gemstones, grab the Fifth Chakra stone and hold it to your Fifth Chakra point on your neck, just below your chin. Imagine it stimulating and strengthening your Fifth Chakra. Imagine your chakra re-calibrating itself to the highly stable vibration of the gemstone, just as a high quality watch keeps accurate time by constantly re-calibrating to the quartz crystal inside it.

ASANAS

Refer to the separate Asana Guide that follows this section. Choose a few and experiment with them. Add more later as you want to, or mix it up as you wish. You can see videos of these asanas at spiralupyoga.com. This book contains seven asanas per chakra. There are many others that you can add as well. See the website for details.

29

SATURDAY: SIXTH CHAKRA DAY

SIXTH CHAKRA OVERVIEW

The Sixth Chakra deals with insight and intuition. The energy of the Sixth Chakra transcends time and space and connects us with deeper wisdom and inspiration. The Sixth Chakra also deals with seeing through surface-level illusions, and strengthening the Sixth Chakra assists us in becoming disillusioned (seeing through illusions) and seeing with greater clarity. The common connotation of being disillusioned is negative, as in being let down or having your expectations shattered. I'd like to invite you to redefine it as I have; seeing through illusions. Understood that way, becoming disillusioned is a wonderful thing and you can feel grateful for anything or anyone that helps you become more disillusioned.

THEME FOR SATURDAYS: SEEING THROUGH ILLUSIONS

Begin all Saturdays with this theme (or choose another phrase from the mantras below, or use your own phrase that fits with the subject matter of the chakra). Make today about noticing all the ways you might be deceived by illusions and how you can see through illusions to a deeper level of truth. All your fears and anxious thinking – are they illusions? If you have strained relationships, what is the illusion that if you could see through it would change how you see things? Let this theme permeate your thinking both while doing specific Spiral Up Yoga practices and throughout the rest of your activities today. With this as your theme, you'll likely be surprised at how many ways you begin to notice illusions and how many things and people become your teachers of this principle of the Sixth Chakra. When the student is ready, the teacher appears. Notice how true this is for you as everything around you becomes a teacher of seeing through illusions and you become the student, really seeing this on many new levels.

The whole world is a form for truth. When someone does not feel grateful to that the forms appear to be as he feels. They mirror his anger, his greed, his fear. Make peace with the universe. Take joy in it. It will turn to gold. Resurrection will be now. Every moment a new beauty.

– RUMI

EMOTIONAL VIBRATION

Focus your thoughts on being connected to the higher intelligence and wisdom of your soul. Imagine a third eye in the center of your brain opening up and able to see with great clarity what is actually going on below the surface of appearances, which can often deceive your physical eyes. See yourself as being inspired by the desires of your soul and guided by your soul's eye to take the next step or two. Trust that the next step is all you ever really need to see, because you have total confidence that your soul will guide you well as you follow your deep desire. Relax and know that your analytical thinking doesn't have to figure everything out and make everything right (not to mention it can't, and usually just makes things worse by trying).

TONING

Sing or tone the word "home," holding out the "om" sound as long as your breath allows. The word "home" both gives the right sound to tone for the Sixth Chakra and has meaning related to the Sixth Chakra. "Home" means trusting that your soul knows the way home and will guide you there. As you hold out the "om" sound, bring your attention to your Sixth Chakra and try to feel it vibrating and glowing. Imagine the deep indigo blue glow getting brighter and stronger.

There is also deep meaning in the "om" sound. The om sound is used in many forms of meditation, prayer, and chanting. It is a fascinating word with deep meaning. Here's my brief summary.

Om comes from Sanskrit and means "the one who protects and sustains order." But its meaning really transcends all language. All languages are made up of words. All words are made up of letters. All letters are really just symbols of sounds. All sounds are just vibrations. Om is a representation of the whole range of vibration. It is really three different sounds blended together: A-U-M.

A is the sound you naturally make by just opening your mouth and making your voice vibrate. U is the sound you naturally make as you round your lips, and M is the sound you naturally make as you close your lips. Try this now and see for yourself. The A and U sounds, blended together, become the O sound and represent the beginning and the middle of all possible sounds. The M sound represents the end of all sound. It is a very calming tone to the brain and is often used to help relax the brain and enter into states of higher awareness. Also, in Sanskrit, the A sound is used to represent the waking state, the U sound the dreaming state, and the M sound the dreamless sleep state. These are the three primary states of being that we all cycle through on a continuous basis.

BREATH

Saturday's breath is called the "alternate-nostril" breath. Here's how you do it:

Any position is fine: standing, sitting, kneeling, or lying on your back. Take a finger and press your left nostril closed, and then inhale deeply through your right nostril and down into your lower abdomen. Then release your left nostril and press your right nostril closed. Exhale slowly and evenly through your left nostril. Now reverse the cycle. Keep your right nostril closed and inhale through your left, then close your left and exhale through your right. Repeat for as many cycles as you want.

The alternate-nostril breath is a very calming and relaxing breath. It stimulates both hemispheres of your brain, as your right nostril is connected to your left brain and your left nostril to your right brain. This breath helps to create a balance of energy in both brain hemispheres. It leads to a relaxed state of awareness that is not unbalanced by over- processing of the left brain (a very common state for most people) or (much less common) an overactive right brain that is not grounded in physical reality. You may find that one side of your nasal passages feels stuffed up and it is more difficult to breathe through that side. If you can get any air through, try to do it, as this will tend to open up the side that is congested. If you can't, that's OK; just do the best you can. Usually one side is open unless you're dealing with a bad sinus cold or infection. You've likely also noticed from personal experience that one side of your nasal passages is congested while the other is open, and which side is open and which congested tends to go back and forth during the day. This is common. I believe it is the result of which side of your brain is currently more active. If the left side is more active, your right nasal passage will be more open, and if the right side of your brain is more active, the left side of your nasal passages will be more open. However, it is quite natural when your Sixth Chakra is open and strong to have both sides of your brain working together and both sides of your nasal passages open and free. The more you practice the alternate-nostril breath and all the other ways of strengthening the Sixth Chakra, the more you will find this to be true for you.

You can do this breath any time during the day: at your desk, sitting in your car, or while watching TV.

EXPERIMENT: ALTERNATE NOSTRIL BREATHING BEFORE & AFTER

As your own personal experiment, try doing alternate nostril breathing before doing your Spiral Up Yoga practice, and notice how clear or blocked is each nostril. Then try again after five minutes or so of your daily practice and see if you notice a difference.

EXPERIMENT Alternate Nostril Breathing Before & After

MANTRA

Here are a few that you could use, or come up with your own that relate to the overall theme of the Sixth Chakra. (To understand the best way to use the mantra, see the discussion of mantras in the "Tools to Strengthen Your Chakras" chapter).

"Seeing through illusions."

"Third eye."

"Deep clarity."

"Insight."

"Soul's guidance."

"Wisdom of not knowing."

ACTIVITIES

- Ask your soul or higher self for guidance and wisdom. Listen for the still, small voice within.

- Pay attention to the pure desires of your heart and trust that this is the most powerful way your soul guides you.

- Surrender to the serenity of not knowing (for now) how everything is going to turn out. Be patient and curious to see how things unfold as you take only the next step that you feel inspired to take.

- Experiment with free writing. Write down a question you have that you don't have the answer to: something that you would like to have more guidance on. Then start writing whatever thoughts you become aware of, no matter what they are, without editing in your head or questioning them.

COLOR GLASSES

If you have purchased a set of chakra color glasses, put on the indigo glasses and see your world through the lens of indigo. Feel it stimulating and resonating with your Sixth Chakra.

TUNING FORK VIBRATION

If you have purchased a set of chakra-calibrated tuning forks, strike the Sixth Chakra tuning fork and place it near your ear. Hum along to the tone, trying to feel the vibration in the Sixth Chakra. Imagine your Sixth Chakra glowing a brighter and stronger indigo (a cross between purple and blue). Strike it again and place the stem on your skull behind your right ear and then again on your skull behind your left ear. Let the vibrations stimulate and permeate both hemispheres of your brain. Next, strike it again and place the stem at the Sixth Chakra point on the centerline of your forehead, about a half inch above your eyebrows. Allow the physical vibration to permeate through your skull and into your brain and imagine it stimulating and strengthening your third eye, or Sixth Chakra.

AROMATHERAPY

If you have purchased a set of chakra-calibrated aromatherapy oils, open the Sixth Chakra vial and inhale the aroma deeply, letting the aroma permeate your entire being. Imagine it stimulating and strengthening your Sixth Chakra. Try covering your left nostril and inhaling through the right nostril, and then reversing and inhaling through the left nostril.

GEMSTONES

If you have purchased a set of chakra gemstones, grab the Sixth Chakra stone and hold it to your Sixth Chakra point, on the centerline of your forehead about a half inch above your eyebrows. Imagine it stimulating and strengthening your Sixth Chakra. Imagine your chakra re-calibrating itself to the highly stable vibration of the gemstone, just as a high quality watch keeps accurate time by constantly re-calibrating to the quartz crystal inside it.

ASANAS

Refer to the separate Asana Guide that follows this section. Choose a few and experiment with them. Add more later as you want to, or mix it up as you wish. You can see videos of these asanas at spiralupyoga.com. This book contains seven asanas per chakra. There are many others that you can add as well. See the website for details.

SUNDAY: SEVENTH CHAKRA DAY

SEVENTH CHAKRA OVERVIEW

The Seventh Chakra deals with spiritual evolution and union with the divine. It symbolizes perfect harmony and complete integration of body, mind, and soul. At the level of the Seventh Chakra, a sense of the separateness of the individual self disappears as the awareness of everything as a perfect unity arises. It is quite limiting to explain the full awakening of any of the chakras with words and logic, but with the Seventh Chakra words and logic are completely inadequate. To be understood, it must be experienced personally. All spiritual concepts of nirvana, heaven, or the promised land are attempts those who have experienced the full awakening of their Seventh Chakras have made to describe what life is like from that state of being.

THEME FOR SUNDAYS: DIVINE PERFECTION

Begin all Sundays with this theme (or choose another phrase from the mantras below, or use your own phrase that fits with the subject matter of the chakra). Make today about noticing all the divine perfection in and around you. Notice how there is perfection even in the things you may have previously seen as flawed or imperfect.

Upgrade your definition of perfection from "no further progress possible," which is how most people see perfection, to "just right for this stage of progress."

For example, look at the life cycle of a tree: from a tiny seed, to a little seedling, to a sprout, to a young tree, to a mature tree with an abundant harvest, to an aged tree, to a dying tree returning to the earth to provide nutrients to other trees. Then ask yourself: "At which stage was the tree not perfect?" What about you? At which stage in your development are you not perfect?

ANALOGY
At Which Stage of Life is the Tree Not Perfect?

Let this theme permeate your thinking both while doing specific Spiral Up Yoga practices and throughout the rest of your activities today. With this as your theme, you'll likely be surprised at how many ways you begin to notice the divine perfection in and around you and how many things and people become your teachers of this principle of the Seventh Chakra. When the student is ready, the teacher appears. Notice how true this is for you as everything around you becomes a teacher of seeing divine perfection and you become the student, really seeing this on many new levels.

Do you think you can take over the universe and improve it?
I do not believe it can be done.
Everything under heaven is a sacred vessel and cannot be controlled.
Trying to control leads to ruin.
Trying to grasp, we lose.

Allow your life to unfold naturally.
Know that it too is a vessel of perfection.
Just as you breathe in and breathe out,
There is a time for being ahead
And a time for being behind;
A time for being in motion
And a time for being at rest;
A time for being vigorous
And a time for being exhausted;
A time for being safe
And a time for being in danger.

To the sage
All of life is a movement toward perfection,
So what need has he
for the excessive, the extravagant or the extreme?
- LAO TZU

EMOTIONAL VIBRATION

Focus your thoughts on your own divinity and eternal nature. Become aware of the fact that you are aware. This awareness has always been with you, regardless of the circumstances of your life. It will always be with you, not just for the rest of your physical life in this body, but forever. What does it feel like to know that you are already immortal, that your awareness is eternal?

TONING

Sing or tone the word "song," holding out the "ong" sound as long as your breath allows. The word "song" both gives the right sound to tone for the Seventh Chakra and has meaning related to the Seventh Chakra. "Song" means becoming one with the great song of all creation: the flowing harmony of celestial being-ness.

There is also deep meaning in the "ong" sound. The "ong" sound comes from Sanskrit and means "creator or the primal vibration from which all creation unfolds." As you hold out the "ong" sound, bring your attention to your Seventh Chakra and try to feel it vibrating and glowing. Imagine a bright purple glow getting brighter and stronger.

Alternatively, some believe the Seventh Chakra is in the realm of silence. So you can silently be for a moment as you focus your attention on the crown of your head until you feel a tingling sensation of energy there.

BREATH

Sunday's breath is called the "heaven and earth" breath. Here's how you do it:

Any position is fine: standing, sitting, kneeling, or lying on your back. Breathe in slowly through your nose (if you can), but imagine that as you breathe in, you are breathing in a pure white light from heaven through the crown of your head and saturating your whole physical and energy body with it. As you breathe out, imagine that you are breathing this energy down through the soles of your feet and into the earth, where it is lovingly accepted and used to nurture the earth. Repeat for as many cycles as you want, feeling the flow of energy from the crown of your head through the soles of your feet.

You can do this breath any time during the day: at your desk, sitting in your car, or while watching TV.

MANTRA

Here are a few that you could use, or come up with your own that relate to the overall theme of the Seventh Chakra. (To understand the best way to use the mantra, see the discussion of mantras in the "Tools to Strengthen Your Chakras" chapter).

"Divine perfection."

"Perfect for this stage of progress."

"I am."

"Eternal truth."

"Perfect unity."

"Heaven and earth are one in me."

ACTIVITIES

- Invite a greater awareness of the divine into your life through ways that inspire you:
    - Listening to inspirational music
    - Meditation
    - Prayer
    - Reading and pondering sacred texts
    - Going to a place of worship
    - Fasting (no food/water for a period of time, and reflection on spiritual things during that time)
    - Taking a walk in nature
    - Playing and laughing with little children
- Do the *I Am* Exercise explained earlier in the *Your Three Bodies* section of the book.

EXPERIMENT: THE "BAD" SOURCE OF ALL YOUR "GOOD"

EXPERIMENT
The "Bad" Source of All Your "Good"

Notice how everything wonderful in your life right now can be traced back to a past event that, when it happened, you didn't think it was so great. And yet because it happened, it put you on the course to experience what you see as wonderful now. Don't make this theoretical. Pick something you love about your life right now and then go back into your past and see how things that happened back then, actually led to creating what you love now. What might that teach you about anything that is currently happening in your life that you see as bad or imperfect?

COLOR GLASSES

If you have purchased a set of chakra color glasses, put on the violet glasses and see your world through the lens of violet. Feel it stimulating and resonating with your Seventh Chakra.

TUNING FORK VIBRATION

If you have purchased a set of chakra-calibrated tuning forks, strike the Seventh Chakra tuning fork and place it near your ear. Hum along to the tone, trying to feel the vibration in the Seventh Chakra. Imagine your Seventh Chakra glowing a brighter and stronger violet/purple. Strike it again and place the stem on your skull behind your right ear and then again on your skull behind your left ear. Let the vibrations stimulate and permeate both hemispheres of your brain. Next, strike it again and place the stem at the Seventh Chakra point on the crown of your head. Allow the physical vibration to permeate through your skull and into your brain, and imagine it stimulating and strengthening your Seventh Chakra.

AROMATHERAPY

If you have purchased a set of chakra-calibrated aromatherapy oils, open the Seventh Chakra vial and inhale the aroma deeply, letting the aroma permeate your entire being. Imagine it stimulating and strengthening your Seventh Chakra. Try covering your left nostril and inhaling through the right nostril, and then reversing and inhaling through the left nostril.

GEMSTONES

If you have purchased a set of chakra gemstones, grab the Seventh Chakra stone and hold it to your Seventh Chakra point, on the crown of your head. Imagine it stimulating and strengthening your Seventh Chakra. Imagine your chakra re-calibrating itself to the highly stable vibration of the gemstone, just as a high quality watch keeps accurate time by constantly re-calibrating to the quartz crystal inside it.

ASANAS

Refer to the separate Asana Guide that follows this section. Choose a few and experiment with them. Add more later as you want to, or mix it up as you wish. You can see videos of these asanas at spiralupyoga.com. This book contains seven asanas per chakra. There are many others that you can add as well. See the website for details.

31

A TYPICAL DAY'S PRACTICE FOR ME

Here's an example of how I personally practice on a typical day. I'm going to pick Monday – First Chakra day.

Soon after awaking and getting out of bed, I take a few deep breaths and remind myself that the overall theme of First Chakra day is "true security within." I use the emotional vibration tool to generate thoughts of being safe, secure, supported, and confident. No matter what comes my way today, I know I can handle it and that my well-being is not ever really at stake. Knowing that, everything else is just an interesting and curious adventure supporting me in my learning and growth. As I am feeling the resulting emotions of being relaxed and confident, I visualize my First Chakra at the root of my torso beginning to gather energy and glow more brightly red, shaking off any accumulated silt. Total time: one minute.

Next I do the mudra lock breath. Total time: one minute.

Next I do a couple of the asanas that I feel like doing.

Total time: one to two minutes. If I feel like it and have time, some days I'll keep doing asanas for five or ten minutes longer.

Then, if I have time, I may go do another form of exercise like running or biking. Even during this other exercise, I try to keep my thoughts gently focused on the theme "true security within." I'm going to be thinking anyway, so why not steer my thinking in that direction?

No extra time involved.

After shaving, showering, and dressing, I stand at my bathroom sink. Next to the sink, where I see them every day, are my aromatherapy oils, tuning forks, color therapy glasses and gemstones. I grab the oil vial for the First Chakra, open it, and deeply inhale the aroma a few times with my eyes closed. I visualize the aroma opening and energizing my First Chakra and a bright red glow emanating from the base of my spine. I then replace the vial and pick up the First Chakra tuning fork, strike it against the striker, and hold it to each ear. I will usually vocalize the First Chakra toning sound ("grow") to the same note as the sound in my ear and focus on feeling the vibration in my First Chakra and seeing the red glow get even stronger. I will then strike the tuning fork again and hold the stem of it against the lower part of my spine at the base of my back. (The First Chakra is the only one that is easier to access from the back of the body than from the front of the body.)

Total time: one to two minutes.

I will then pretty much go about my day, doing whatever I do. In the back of my mind I'll be remembering the theme of the day (true security within) and recalling it as needed when I may start to feel insecure or fearful about something. I'll remind myself, "Worst case, it won't go the way I want, and I'll learn something and my well-being is still intact. Best case, it will go the way I want, and I'll learn something and my well-being is still intact." There may be times during the day where I find myself getting a little agitated and insecure. This is a good time to start silently repeating my favorite mantra for the day, which might be the same as the theme: "True security within. True security within …"

After dinner, I will typically play with the younger kids in the backyard. I'll take my shoes and socks off and go barefoot and play in the grass or over in the sand area. Walking barefoot in nature is one of the simple activities that helps strengthen the First Chakra, as I am making direct physical contact with the earth and my sole chakras. I would be playing outside with the kids anyway, so no additional time is required, just a shift in awareness.

At night, after the kids are in bed and I've got a little time before going to bed, I may sit with my wife and watch a show we both enjoy. While watching it, I may sit on the ground instead of the couch and do a few more asanas.

There is no extra time involved. This is bonus time, since I'm still watching TV, which I would have been doing anyway.

Then, right before going to bed, I will often do another minute with the aromatherapy oil and the tuning fork. Total time: one minute.

So you can see it's really just a minute or two here and there, and it just fits simply into my day. Notice that I never had to change into special clothes (most of it I did in my pj's), pull out a special mat, put on a special DVD, arrange my schedule around a specific class time, or drive anywhere.

Really, the only parts that need to be learned are the asanas. At the beginning, if you've never done yoga before, it will take some time to get familiar with them, but they are fun and interesting to learn, and it feels great to do them. The images of the asanas in this book can be referred to as often as needed. Additionally, there will be videos available on spiralupyoga.com, and large-format wall charts that can be purchased for easy reference. Eventually we even plan to offer a mobile phone app, so even when you're traveling you can have the reference materials at your fingertips.

32
CREATING YOUR OWN PRACTICE: TEST, THEN TRUST

The Spiral Up Yoga system is designed to be highly customizable. The whole point is to make it something that you want to do for a few minutes every day because of what it does for you. I've developed a high level of trust in my own practice of the system, and I am constantly changing it up from day to day and week to week. No two days are the same, and no two weeks are the same. But my trust came from testing it out and experimenting with how it made me feel both in the moment and in general, over time.

So my suggestion to you is this: don't trust this system (that will come later). Test it. Try a little bit of this and a little bit of that. Try a few asanas, try the breath work, try the toning, try the aromatherapy, try the tuning forks, try it all. There's no rush. This is a lifelong foundational practice you're creating, and it will truly be your own creation. I've just provided some foundational understanding, a simple, flexible structure, and some tools and methods that I have found work effectively. As you test it and begin to experience your own results, you'll begin to develop trust in it, and it will truly become your own foundation for daily self-care of body, mind, and soul.

You may even come up with your own additional tools or practices that help you to open and strengthen your chakras. As you do, please feel free to share them with other practitioners of Spiral Up Yoga on our website. I invite you to become an active member of the Spiral Up Yoga worldwide tribe where you can support and be supported by others.

What we hope ever to do with ease, we must first learn to do with diligence.
– SAMUEL JOHNSON

Those who offer instant enlightenment mislead us. After all, we have to bring the mind itself under control, and there is no more difficult task in life. We should be prepared for a lifetime of challenge. But then, we need challenges, or we stagnate. If you want to judge your progress, ask yourself these questions: Am I more loving? Is my judgment sounder? Do I have more energy? Can my mind remain calm under provocation? Am I free from the conditioning of anger, fear, and greed? Spiritual awareness reveals itself eloquently in character development and selfless action. Authentic spiritual experience changes the way you see the world and the way you live.
- EKNATH EASWAREN

T.T.T.
Put up in a place
Where it's easy to see
The cryptic admonishment
-T.T.T.

When you feel how depressingly
Slowly you climb,
It's well to remember that
Things Take Time
- PIET HEIN

Nibble at me.
Don't gulp me down.
How often is it you have a guest in your house
Who can fix everything?
- RUMI

THE ENDLESS HORIZON AHEAD

No matter how far you walk, the horizon ahead of you will always look just as far away. To have a sense of progress, you must look back and notice how far you've come; otherwise, you'll likely become discouraged if you only focus on how much more progress there is to make. Be patient with yourself. Spiral Up Yoga is not a *quick-fix* program; it is a *deep-fix* practice. Once you begin, you will notice some of the benefits pretty quickly, and those benefits will continue to accrue as you continue to practice for just a few minutes on a daily basis. Ultimately, Spiral Up Yoga is the true fix for everything because it is really a daily, incremental restoration of your own innate divinity and power of body, mind, and soul.

Remember, it is a lifelong practice, not a ninety-day exercise regimen. There is no finish line, but there are many signs of progress that you'll be able to notice on many levels of body, mind and soul. If it ever seems like your progress is too slow and you begin to get frustrated, use the wisdom contained in these quotes to remind yourself that you're doing just fine. If you do get frustrated, ask yourself which part of you is frustrated – the personality or the soul? Then calmly reassure your personality that each little bit of chakra opening and strengthening that you do is for its benefit too, and do one or two of your Spiral Up Yoga practices for just five minutes (or even less). The horizon looks just as far ahead of you as always, but you've moved forward in a meaningful way in just those few minutes.

THE ASANAS

The following are the asanas I have chosen to include in this book. I have chosen seven asanas for each of the seven chakras. While there are hundreds, maybe even thousands of yoga asanas, I have specifically chosen these because they are very effective in opening and strengthening the particular chakra they are listed under. I have generally chosen asanas that are easier to do for beginners, but still allow a wide range of depth so that even those who are more experienced practitioners of yoga can remain challenged. I'm not into doing the "human pretzel" asanas. This isn't about showing off how flexible you are, it's about building a solid foundation of daily chakra opening and strengthening that is accessible to all people regardless of experience level with yoga. I have included a few more challenging asanas so you have something to work towards. Don't worry if you can't do them as the pictures and description show. Just do the best you can from where you're at today and know that as you keep doing these, you will definitely improve your flexibility, strength, and balance.

This section of the book contains photos and descriptions of the asanas, but you can also go to our website www.spiralupyoga.com and watch brief videos on each asana to get a better feel for it. Some of the asanas involve a lot of motion, and video does a much better job of showing that. The videos for the forty-nine asanas contained in this book are available to view for free on our website.

In many cases, I have used traditional names (in English) for these asanas, and practitioners of yoga will recognize some of the names. I don't like using the Sanscrit names since many are difficult to pronounce and remember. For whatever reason, yoga instructors often like to use these names, but I prefer English names that are somewhat descriptive of the asana itself, and they are easy to remember by name once you've done them a few times. In other cases, I have used my own names that just seem to describe the asana better. You can call them by your own names if you come up with a better name for you. The name isn't important; the asana is.

A few guidelines that apply to doing any of the asanas:

1. If you have any medical conditions or limitations, please consult with your doctor and use your own wisdom. I am not a medical doctor and don't give medical advice. These asanas can help you increase the flexibility, strength and balance of your physical body, as well as improve your mindfulness and your connection with your soul, but please be gentle and patient with your body (and mind).

Remember, it is not about intensity, but about small and simple repeated consistently. Don't worry if you can't do them as shown in the pictures. Just do them the best you can from where you're at right now. and trust that you will improve over time.

2. You don't need to do all seven asanas every day. You certainly can if you want to, but all you really need to maintain a solid foundation is just picking a few of them, even just one or two each day. There may be some days when you'll want to do all of them, and spend longer doing each one. There will be other days when you may only fit one in for thirty seconds. There may even be a few days when you don't do any, but you still remember to do some of the other chakra strengthening tools such as breath work, aromatherapy oils, or tuning forks. It's all good.

3. It is always best to do asanas on an empty stomach, so plan accordingly. It's fine if you've just had a glass of water or a piece of fruit, but if you've just eaten a full meal, it's best to wait for an hour or more before doing asanas. It's also good to be well hydrated before and after doing asanas. Drink a small amount of room temperature water (not cold water) before doing your asanas, and then drink plenty of water after, as it will help to flush the toxins you have literally squeezed from your organs and tissues during your asana work.

4. In addition to doing the physical asanas, a big part of the effectiveness comes from also including mindful presence and conscious breathing while you do the asanas. This means bringing your full attention to your asanas and your breath while you do them. Let the sound of your breath and the beat of your heart be the music you listen to as you perform your daily asanas. This is how you know you are fully present.

5. Much of the breath work you do during your asana work will feel intuitive and natural. In most cases, I explain the best breath structure for each asana. In some cases, I will refer to something called "The Breath of Fire," which is a specific energizing breath outlined earlier in the breath work section (Wednesday, Third Chakra day). The Breath of Fire is something that will be utilized during asana work on any day (not just Wednesdays). To review, it is a fairly rapid in/out breath through the nose and into the belly. Two in/out cycles per second is about the right speed.

6. If you feel any sharp pain while doing an asana, back off and ease up. It's fine, and even good, to feel a little discomfort as you stretch your body that has become compressed and tight and begin to open in up again. The asanas are designed to take your body out of its comfort zone and into a stretching zone, but not so far that you injure a body part. So find your own zone of stretching a bit past your

comfort zone, but don't push it too far. Tiny, small steps consistently over time are much more transformative than willful intensity.

7. Pay attention to how you feel before vs. after doing your asana work. Compare things such as your energy level, your level of alertness, how tight or loose you feel in your body, how calm or agitated your mind is, and how peaceful you feel. Notice if your mouth feels dry or moist. Notice if your breathing feels constricted or open. This mindful checking in with your body, mind and soul both before and after doing asana work will give you your own personal experience and "proof" of the effectiveness of this work completely independent of anything I say or claim in this book. The way just a few minutes each day of this asana work can make you feel will hopefully give you all the inspiration you need to continue doing it every day. Ultimately enjoying the process and the immediate result is what will make this sustainable for you. Don't worry about an end result or a timetable of progress; there is no final stopping place or timetable. This is a lifelong self-care practice that will evolve and change with you.

The following pictures and descriptions explain how to do the asanas. It will likely be helpful to also watch the brief videos of each asana available on the website www.spiralupyoga.com when first learning these asanas. Once you've learned them, referring to the pictures will usually be enough. After a while, just reading the name of the asana will be enough for you to know what to do. Eventually, you'll just have your favorites and you'll know what to do without referring to anything.

ASANA 1-1: Base Pump

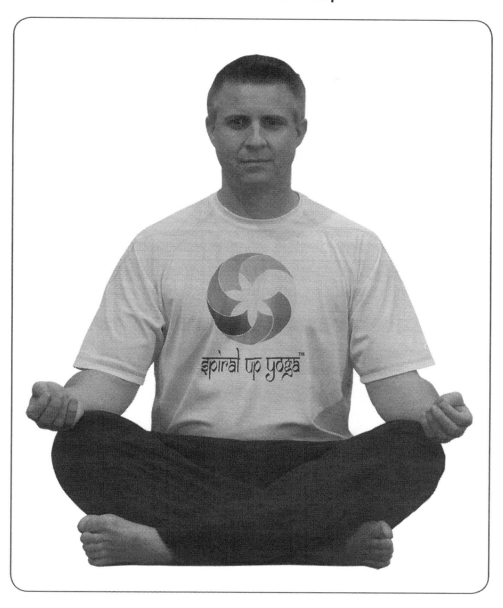

Sit in a cross-legged position with hands resting on knees as shown (Figure 1). Now begin squeezing all your lower torso muscles from your anus to your navel. Squeeze in and hold one to two seconds and then release. Repeat this squeeze and release pump action for thirty to sixty seconds. This stimulates and strengthens your First Chakra. Breathe naturally as you do this, and don't worry about trying to time your breath with your squeezing and releasing. You can do this anytime during the day when sitting at your desk or on your couch.

ASANA 1-2: Seated Pelvic Rotations

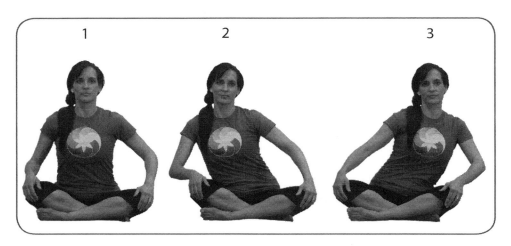

Sit in a cross-legged position. Grab your knees with your hands (Figure 1). Begin slowly rotating your hips and waist in a clockwise circle. Imagine your navel is tracing as wide a circle around your seated center position as possible. Use your arms as leverage (Figures 2 and 3). Keep the movement slow and steady, breathing naturally and without trying to synchronize your breath with your movement. Breathe through your nose if you can. Continue this clockwise movement for twenty to thirty seconds. Now reverse the direction and begin rotating in a counter clockwise direction for another twenty to thirty seconds.

ASANA 1-3: Crow

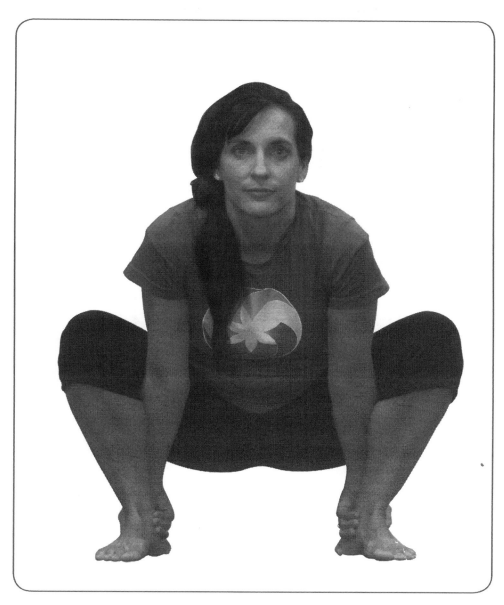

Begin standing with feet set wider than shoulders. Squat down and place arms in front of thighs, reaching around to grab the heels of your feet, or resting your fingertips on the floor behind your heels to maintain balance (Figure 1). Keep your head up looking forward. Do the Breath of Fire through your nose, pumping air from the lower abdomen area at a quicker than normal pace. Two in/out breaths per second is a good pace. Hold this position for as long as you want; usually about twenty to sixty seconds is fine.

ASANA 1-4: Namaste Squat

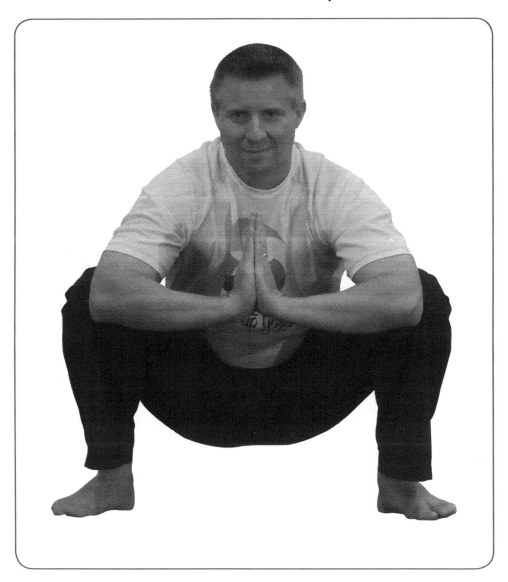

Begin standing with feet set wider than shoulders. Squat down and place elbows on the inside of each knee. Place palms of hands together in the Namaste position. Keep your head up looking forward (Figure 1). Do the Breath of Fire through your nose, pumping air from lower abdomen area at a quicker than normal pace. Two in/out breaths per second is a good pace. Hold this position for as long as you want; usually about twenty to sixty seconds is fine.

ASANA 1-5: Wide Angle Forward Bend

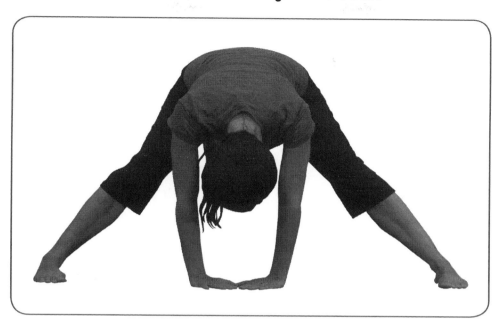

Begin in a standing position. Spread legs wide apart, toes pointing straight ahead. Keep knees straight and bend forward from the hips, placing hands on the floor between your feet. If you can, place your palms flat on the floor. Head is looking down at the floor (Figure 1). Breathing is long deep breathing from lower abdomen. Hold this position for as long as you want; usually twenty to sixty seconds is fine. Slowly come back up to standing and walk feet back to hip width distance.

ASANA 1-6: Crouching Ninja

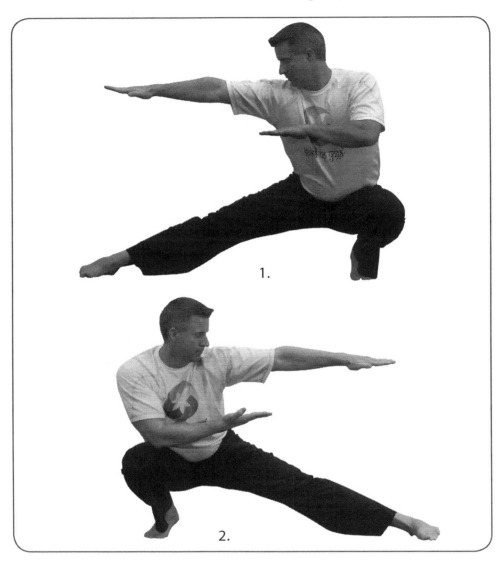

1.

2.

Begin in standing position. Step feet wide apart, toes pointing forward. Slowly crouch down to one side, bending the knee on that side and raising the heel up. On the other side, straighten the leg and knee and keep that foot firmly planted on the ground, toes still pointing forward. Place arms/hands pointing in the direction of the straight leg and look in that direction (Figure 1). Hold this position for a few counts while breathing naturally through nose. Now slowly reverse direction doing the same thing, but on the other side (Figure 2). You will rise up a little and then back down again as you move to the other side. Go back and forth from one side to the other in a slow, smooth motion. Continue this back and forth motion as long as you like; usually thirty to sixty seconds is fine.

ASANA 1-7: Karate Kicks

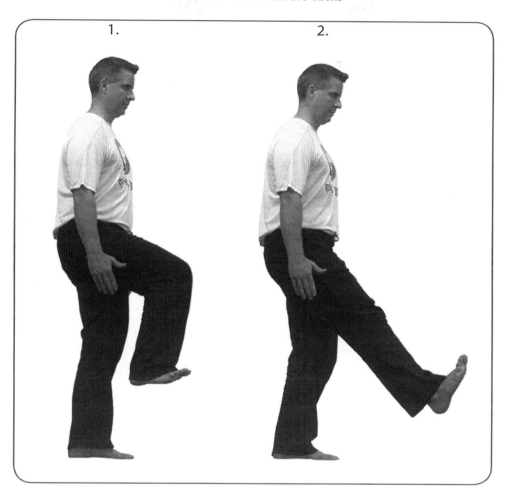

Begin in a standing position. Lift one leg/knee up and balance on the other foot. Toe should be pointing up, heel stretched down (Figure 1). If you need to hold onto a wall or table to do this, that's fine. Next, with energy, extend your lifted leg forward and out, straightening your lifted leg and pointing your heel as if striking and breaking a board with your heel (Figure 2). Imagine sending energy from your core through your leg and out your heel. Breathe out loudly through your mouth as you strike forward with your heel, making an audible "haaaa" sound. Repeat on the other side. Go back and forth from side to side for as long as you want; usually twenty to sixty seconds is fine.

ASANA 2-1: Hula Hips

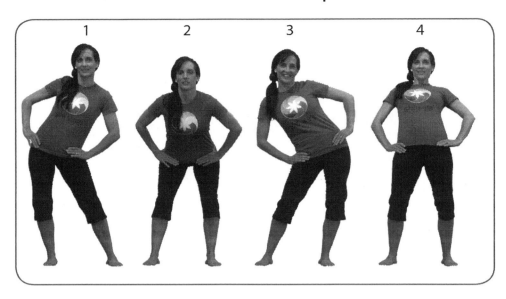

Begin in the standing position, feet a bit wider than shoulder width apart, toes pointing forward. Place your hands on your hips and slowly rotate your hips in a clockwise direction, making as large a circle around your centerline as you can while keeping your feet planted (Figures 1,2,3,4). Breathe naturally as you rotate for twenty to thirty seconds in a clockwise direction and then reverse to a counter-clockwise direction for another twenty to thirty seconds. Imagine the circumference of your hip circle being drawn in bright orange by your Second Chakra.

ASANA 2-2: Lower Spinal Flex

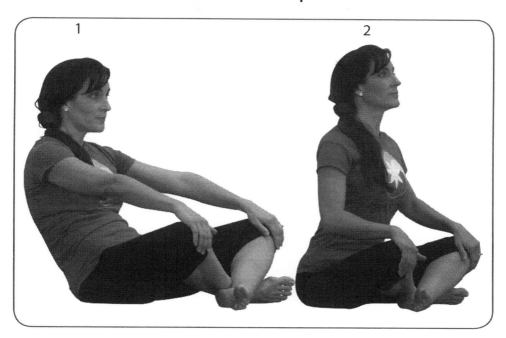

Begin in a cross-legged seated position. Place your hands over your knees (or alternatively place hands in front of ankles). Begin a back and forth movement, flexing your lower spine back and forth (Figures 1 and 2). Breathe in as you flex forward and out as you flex back. Continue movement as long as you like; usually twenty to sixty seconds is fine.

ASANA 2-3: Seated Forward Fold

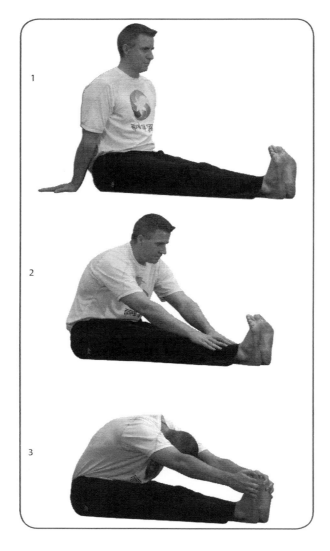

Begin in a seated position with your legs straight in front and your feet together, toes pulled back toward your body, heels flexed (Figure 1). Gently lean forward and reach as far as you can towards your feet while keeping your knees locked and your legs straight (Figure 2). Relax your neck and drop your head so you are looking down at your knees. As your head drops, lower it toward your knees (Figure 3). As your flexibility grows, you will be able to reach further and touch your toes, and eventually you'll be able to hold the soles of your feet. You may want to begin a gentle bouncing motion when you reach the extent of your current flexibility. Do this by moving back and forth an inch or two in a gentle bounce. As you hold the stretch, breathe long slow breaths, consciously relaxing your hamstrings and lower back muscles. Hold the position at the edge of your current flexibility (just slightly past your comfort zone) for as long as you like; usually ten to thirty seconds is fine.

ASANA 2-4: Layback Between Heels

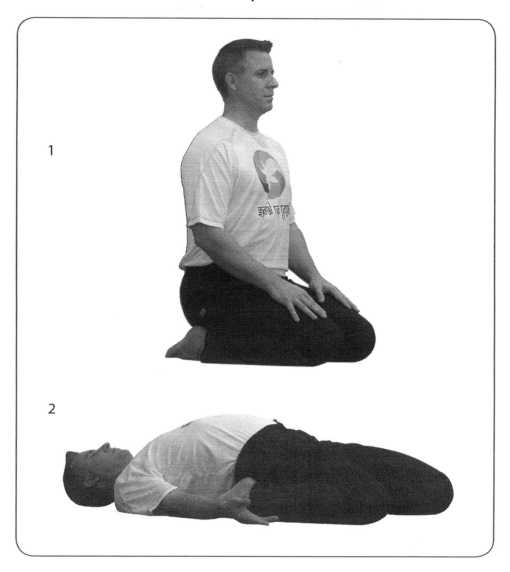

Begin in a kneeling position, sitting between your heels (Figure 1). Slowly lean back, keeping your seat between your heels until your head and back is resting on the floor with your arms resting at your side (Figure 2). You can stay in this position as long as you like, breathing long slow breaths from the lower abdomen, usually twenty to sixty seconds is fine. Only go back as far as you can for now. You can support your weight with your hands or forearms behind you on the floor. As you increase in flexibility you will be able to lay completely back with your head and back touching the floor, and your arms resting at your sides.

ASANA 2-5: Hip Raises

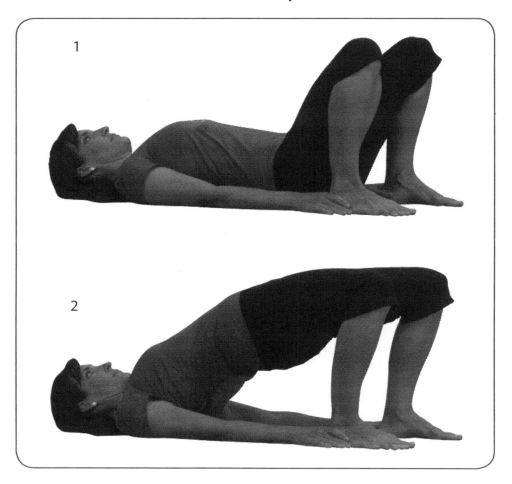

Begin by lying on your back and pulling your heels toward your hips (Figure 1). Grab your heels with your hands and then raise your hips and back off the ground and up so that your shoulders and feet are supporting your weight (Figure 2). Repeat this motion, raising and lowering your hips and back, for as long as you like; usually twenty to sixty seconds is fine. Breathe in as you rise up and out as you lower back down.

ASANA 2-6: Locust

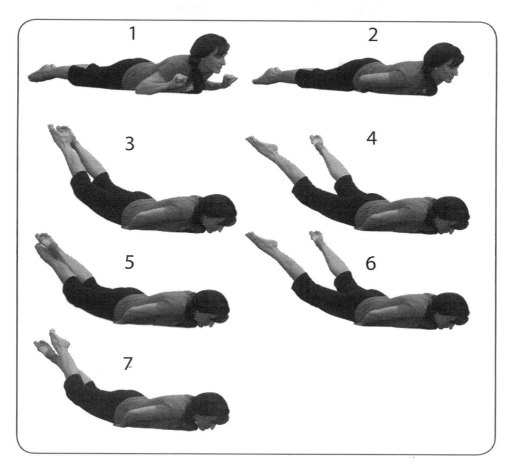

Begin by lying on your front, legs extended, toes pointing back (Figure 1). Make your hands into fists and place them under your hip bones (Figure 2). Place your chin on the floor and lift both legs up behind you; your weight should be supported by your hips/fists and your chin (Figure 3). With your legs lifted, begin moving them out (Figure 4) and back in crossing at the ankles (Figure 5) and then out again (Figure 6) and in again, reversing the cross of the ankles (Figure 7). Continue this out/in motion reversing the cross of the ankles with each repetition. Continue for as long as you like; usually ten to thirty seconds is fine. Do the Breath of Fire as you do this asana (rapid in/out through your nose, two ins, two outs per second is about the right pace).

ASANA 2-7: Camel

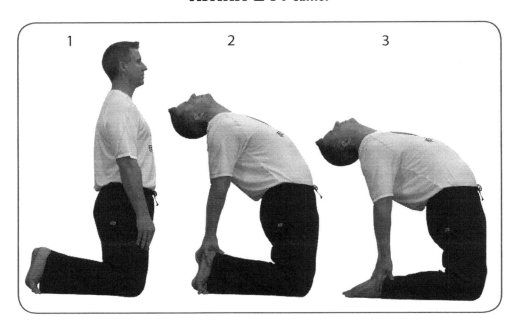

Begin kneeling, toes pointed under, thighs straight up (Figure 1). Slowly bend backwards, grabbing your heels with your hands to support yourself. Drop your head back so your neck is stretched and you are looking up and back (Figure 2). As you progress, you may be able to lower your feet so they are flat on the ground (Figure 3). Hold your position for as long as you like; usually ten to thirty seconds is fine. Do long deep breathing through nose while you hold your position. When done, slowly ease back up into the kneeling upright position you started with.

ASANA 3-1: Four-Way Bends

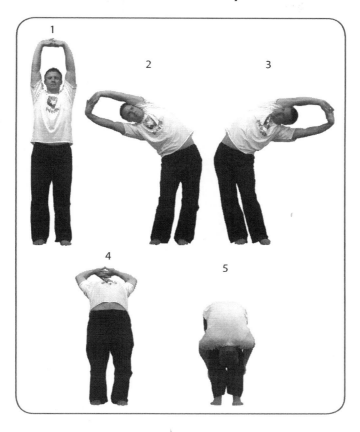

Begin in a standing position, legs hip width apart. Interlock your fingers then invert your hands so your palms are facing toward the sky. Stretch your arms up above your head and extend them as far as you can, really pulling them up so that your biceps are touching your ears (Figure 1). Now bend to your left, maintaining a full stretch along the outside of your body, from toes to hands. Your right bicep should be touching your right ear as you bend and stretch to the left and your right hip comes out to the right (Figure 2). Hold this position for a few counts and really feel the meridian stretch along the entire right side of your body from lower leg to your right pinky finger. Now reverse and do the same thing on the left side – left hip moves out to left, left bicep on left ear (Figure 3). Return to center position, while keep arms above head. Now gently lean backwards, eyes looking at your knuckles. Feel the stretch in the entire front body (Figure 4). Return to center and drop arms, placing your hands at your lower back, as if your palms are covering up your kidneys. Take a slight backward bend and then gently bend forward, dropping your head and upper body into a forward fold as your arms and hands slide down the back of your legs to provide support and leverage to pull down as far as you are able right now (Figure 5). Feel the stretch in your back body and hold for several counts and then slowly rise back up to a rested standing position. Imagine your solar plexus as the center of gravity around which you are stretching in all directions. This is a great one that stretches and opens all your meridians – front, back, left and right sides.

ASANA 3-2: Starfish

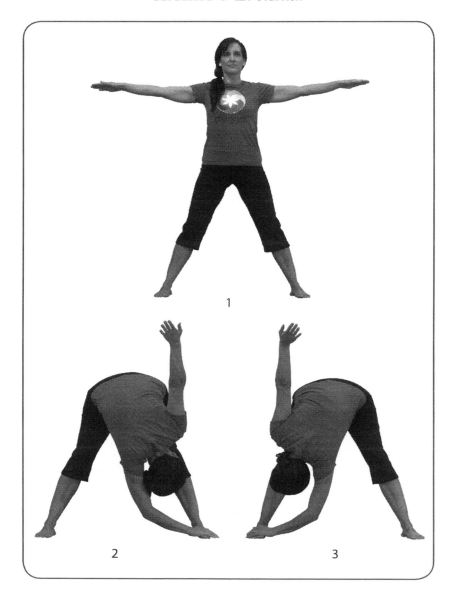

Begin in a standing position – legs set wide apart, feet pointing forward and arms stretched straight out to sides, palms down. You will look a bit like a starfish (Figure 1). Now twist your upper body to the left and bend forward towards your left foot, with your head dropping toward your body. Your right arm reaches toward your left foot and your left arm raises up behind you (Figure 2). Return to the starting position and do the same thing on the right side (Figure 3). Return to starting position and repeat, going back and forth between left and right sides several times. Breathe out as you go down and in as you come back up. Make the motions smooth and slow, not fast and jerky. Twist your upper body first and then bend forward to go down.

ASANA 3-3: The Washing Machine

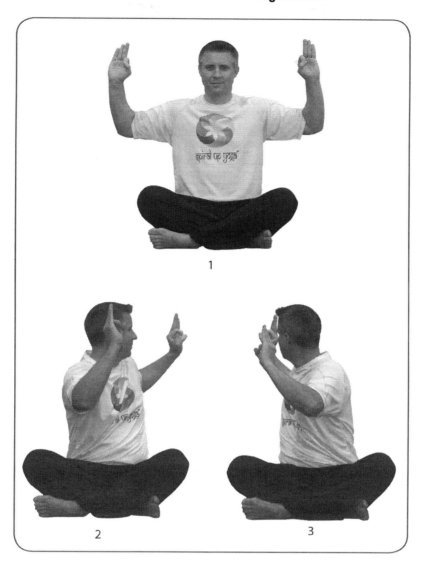

Sit in a cross-legged position. Raise both your arms to the square (90 degree or so angle at the elbow). Touch thumb to first finger, leaving the other three fingers extended (Figure 1). Now begin twisting your upper body back and forth from left to right, breathing out as you go to either side and in as you move back through center. Allow your head and neck to twist with your body so the whole upper body is moving as one unit, twisting at the waist (Figures 2 and 3). Keep this back and forth motion going for twenty to sixty seconds. You can start slow and increase speed as you go. This is meant to be done with energy and speed. Imagine you are a washing machine gyrating back and forth, cleansing your liver of toxins as you do (which is exactly what you are doing; you are literally squeezing your liver like you would squeeze the dirty water out of a sponge).

ASANA 3-4: Boat

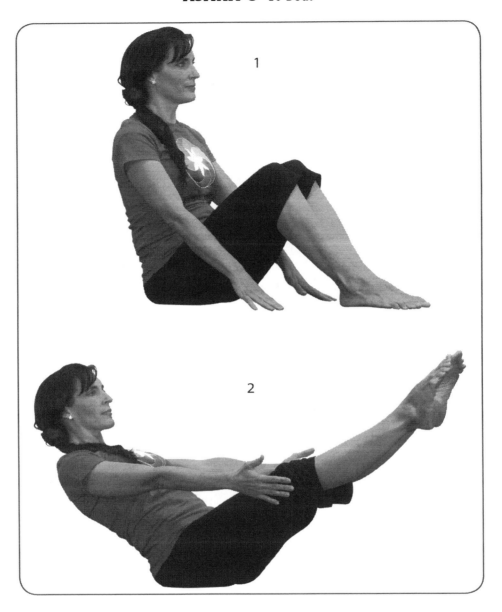

This is a balancing pose that really stimulates the Third Chakra. Begin in a seated position, with feet flat on floor, knees bent. Lean your upper body back slightly (Figure 1). Now slowly raise your legs, with your feet pointed and keeping your legs as straight as you can. You may place your hands palm down on the ground for balance and support or if you can, raise your hands off the ground and straighten your arms forward, palms facing each other and balancing completely on your sit bones (Figure 2). Hold this position for a few counts, breathing the Breath of Fire as you hold. Lower your feet and hands when done. Repeat if you like.

ASANA 3-5: Stretch Pose

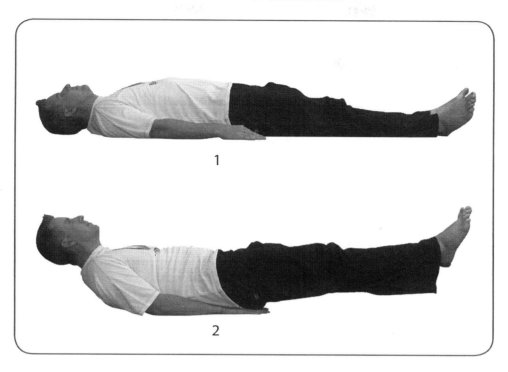

1

2

This is another balancing pose that is great for the Third Chakra. Lie on your back and place your hands, palms down, beneath your hips. This will form your balance point and support your lower back (Figure 1). Now lift both legs with toes pointing forward and also lift your head and upper body with your head and neck stretching back, away from your feet (Figure 2). You'll want to feel a good stretch from head to toe. Hold this pose for ten to thirty seconds, doing the Breath of Fire as you hold.

ASANA 3-6: Forearm Alternating Leg Lifts

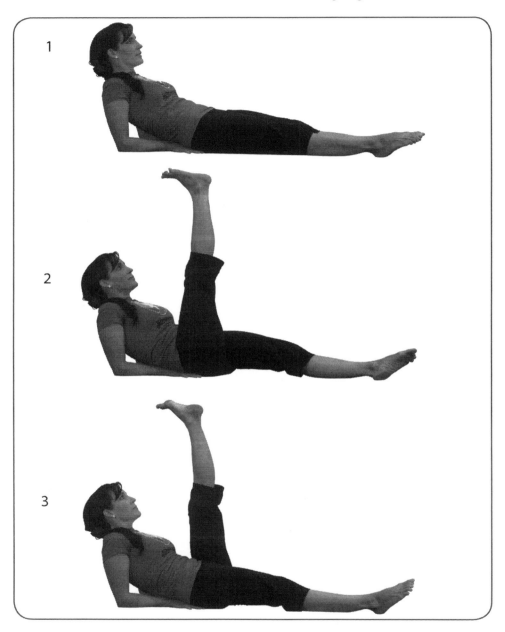

Begin by lying on your back with your legs flat on the ground and your arms to your sides. Now raise your upper body and rest on your forearms, palms down, head forward, looking towards toes (Figure 1). From here, raise one leg up and back, keeping the leg straight as you do with the toes pulled back towards your shin and heel extended (Figure 2). Then lower that leg with the toes now pointing forward, and repeat with the other leg (Figure 3). Go back and forth, alternating the leg lifts. Breathe in as you raise a leg and out as you lower it. Continue for twenty to sixty seconds.

ASANA 3-7: Bow

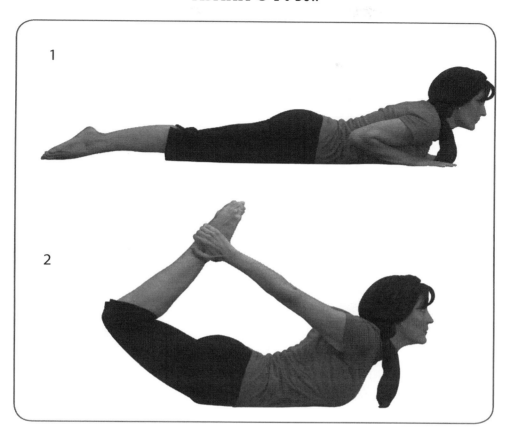

This one is a little more advanced. If you're just beginning, just take this gently and don't worry if you can't do it well yet; you will before long. Begin by lying on your front. Place your palms flat on the ground near your chest as if you were going to do a push up (Figure 1). Now raise your lower legs up at the knees and reach your arms back and grab your ankles. Once you have a firm hold on your ankles, pull your ankles forwards, raising your thighs off the ground and raising your upper body off the ground with your head looking forward (Figure 2). You can extend the stretch by also bending your neck and head back so you are looking up. Hold this position for several counts – usually ten to thirty seconds. Release your ankles and return to lying position.

ASANA 4-1: Under Arrest

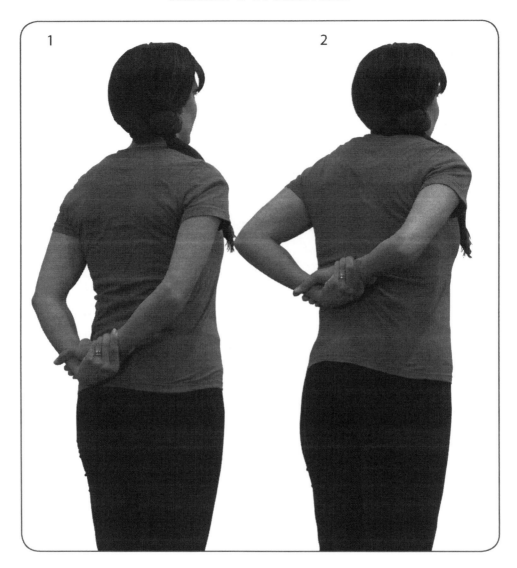

Begin in a standing position. Place arms behind back with wrists along the line of the spine at your lower back. Grab one wrist with the other hand, almost like your hands are tied behind your back (Figure 1). Now slowly pull your hands up the line of your spine and back down again as if you are trying to get your hands loose from the binding (Figure 2). Your shoulders should move forward and then back in a circular motion as your hands move up and then back down your spine. Breath in as you move hands up the spine, and out as they move back down. Repeat for twenty to sixty seconds.

ASANA 4-2: Heart Bow

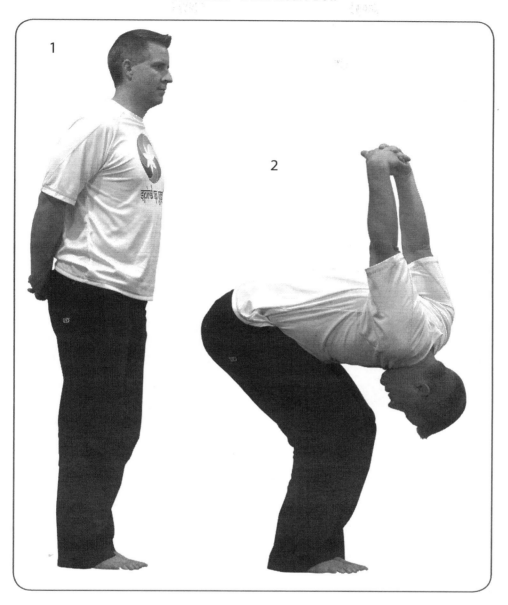

Begin in a standing position, feet together, place hands behind back, interlocking the fingers (Figure 1). Now bend your knees and drop your head towards your knees while you pull back and up with your arms, raising them up above your head (Figure 2). Feel the stretch across your chest, shoulders and arms. Hold for as long as you like; about ten to thirty seconds is plenty, and return to the beginning position. Long, deep breathing as you hold this pose, feeling your Fourth Chakra (heart center) opening.

ASANA 4-3: Cobra

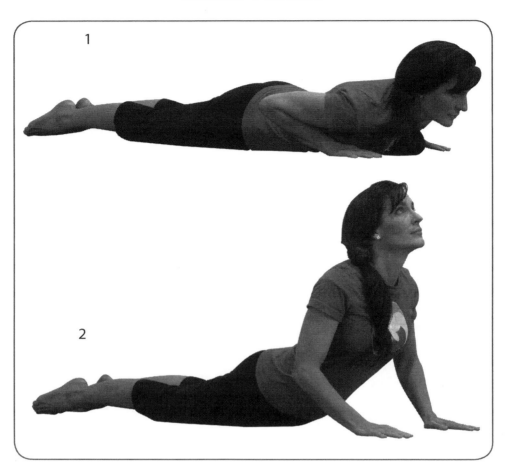

Begin by lying on your front. Place your hands palms down, near your shoulders, like you are about to do a push up, but toes are pointing away from you, with the front of your feet flat on the floor (Figure 1). Support your weight on your hands and lower legs as you pull your upper body off the ground. Pull up from your torso, not really with your hands and arms, which are just there to support you (Figure 2). Feel the stretch in your lower back and in your Fourth Chakra heart center. You can either look forward as you hold this pose, or extend your neck and head back to extend the upper body stretch. Hold for as long as you like – about ten to thirty seconds is plenty – while doing long, deep breathing, and then return to the beginning position.

ASANA 4-4: Venus Fly Trap

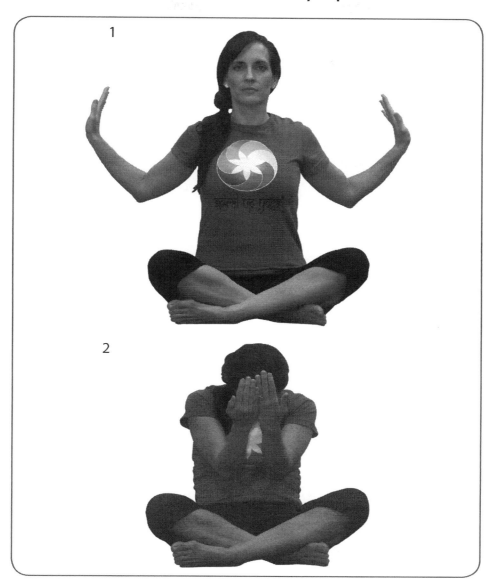

Begin seated cross-legged. Raise your arms so that your hands are about at eye level, palms facing toward your eyes, with pinky fingers touching each other. Now pull your elbows and shoulders back as you open your front body, feeling a stretch in your chest area. Flex your upper body and spine forward as you pull your arms back, then reverse, closing your arms in front of you and flexing your upper body and spine backwards (Figures 1 and 2). Imagine you are a Venus fly trap plant, opening up wide and waiting for a fly to land and then closing up tightly to trap the fly. Continue this opening and closing motion for as long as you like; twenty to thirty seconds is plenty. Breathe in as you open up and out as you close.

ASANA 4-5: Sliding Doors

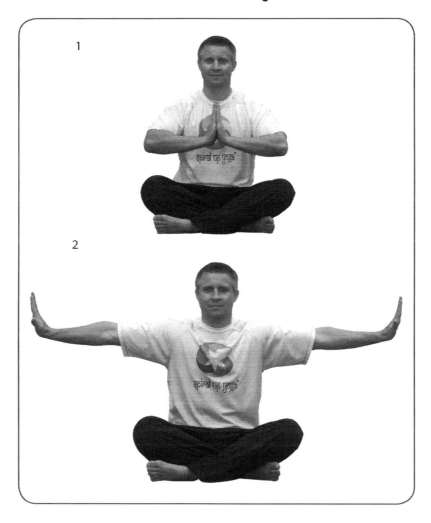

Begin seated cross-legged. Hold your hands palms together (Namaste mudra) at your Fourth Chakra (Figure 1). Now, with force, thrust your arms out from the center to each side simultaneously, like a sliding glass door that opens from the center to both sides. Send energy from your Fourth Chakra all the way down both arms and out the palms of each hand. In the open position, your arms should be fully extended to each side, your elbows straight and your palms facing away from you, and your hands at a ninety-degree angle to your arms (Figure 2). Begin a rather rapid back and forth motion, bringing the palms together and clapping them right in front of your Fourth Chakra and then pressing them out with force to the fully open and extended position. Keep this open, close motion going rapidly for twenty to sixty seconds. Focus on breathing out with force through your nose as you extend your arms out, almost like doing a karate chop to a board with the balls of your hands. You will naturally breathe in as you close. If you want to challenge yourself one day, try doing this for two to three minutes without stopping.

ASANA 4-6: Alternating Bridge/Staff

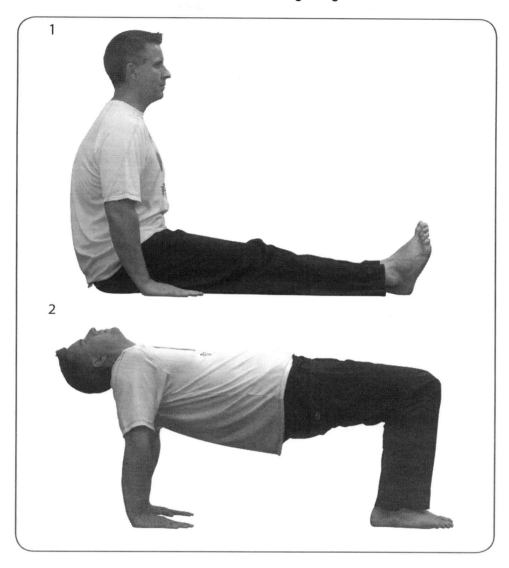

Begin seated with legs extended in front of your feet about shoulder width apart. Hands are palms down, slightly behind your hips with fingers pointing forward (Figure 1). From this position (Staff), press up onto your palms and feet, letting your head drop back into Bridge position (Figure 2). From this position you should feel a good stretch across your Fourth Chakra. Your front body, hips and thighs should be fairly level, like a bridge. Now return back to the first position. Repeat this down and up motion, moving between positions gently, and slowly. If you'd like to, begin increasing the speed with which you move back and forth between positions. Continue for as long as you like; usually twenty to sixty seconds is plenty. Breathe in as you move up into Bridge and out as you move down into Staff.

ASANA 4-7: Alternating Up/Down Dog

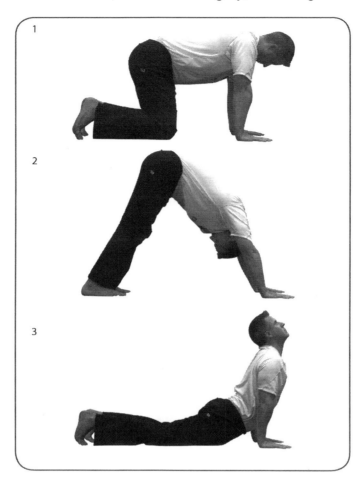

Begin in a kneeling position, knees below hips and also with hands, palm down on the ground with wrists below shoulders (Figure 1). From here, press up into Down Dog position (Figure 2). In this position, your legs are straight, knees locked, and your feet are flat on the floor. Your butt is in the air and your head is down towards the floor with a relaxed neck, looking back at your knees. Your elbows are also locked, arms straight. You should be forming an upside-down V at this point. You may not be able to keep your feet flat at first; that's something you'll eventually work into. Don't worry if your heels come off the floor or your knees don't lock. From here, keep your toes and hands in place as you move your butt from the top to the bottom and your head and upper torso come up into Up Dog position (Figure 3). At this point all your weight is on your hands and toes and your upper body is stretched back and your neck and head are stretched back as you look up towards the ceiling/sky. Get a good feel for these two positions and then begin moving back and forth between them, at first slowly, and then with more speed. Breathe in as you move into Up Dog (Figure 3) and out as you move into Down Dog (Position 2). Continue this up/down motion for twenty to sixty seconds.

ASANA 5-1: Shoulder Circles

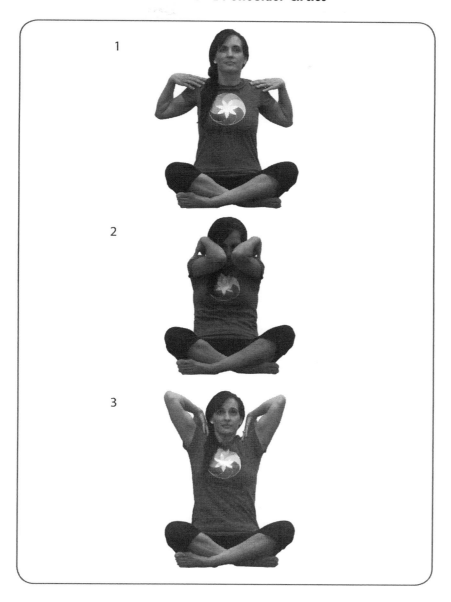

Begin seated cross-legged. Place your hands on your shoulders with your fingers in front and your thumb on back (Figure 1). While holding your hands in that position, begin rotating your arms down and towards each other until they touch at your center line (Figure 2). Keep rotating in a large circular motion so that your elbows are now above your head and your biceps are touching your ears (Figure 3). Keep the circular motion going and bring your elbows back down and around. Keep repeating this circular motion for as many repetitions as you want. Flex your upper spine back and forth as you make these circular motions with your arms. Breathe in as your elbows go back and up and your chest is expanded and out as your spine flexes back and your elbows come down.

ASANA 5-2: Towel Wringing

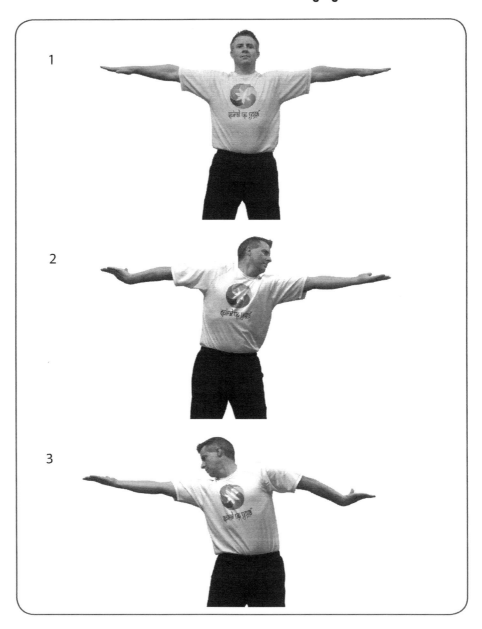

1

2

3

Begin in a standing position, feet shoulder width apart. Extend both arms out to the sides, palms facing down (Figure 1). Now, begin twisting your arms and shoulders as if they were a long towel that you are wringing water out of. Turn your head to the left as you rotate your palms from downward facing to upward facing (Figure 2). Then turn your head to the right as you rotate your palms 360 degrees from back to upward facing again (Figure 3). Keep going back and forth like this for as long as you like; usually twenty to sixty seconds is fine.

ASANA 5-3: Head Rolls

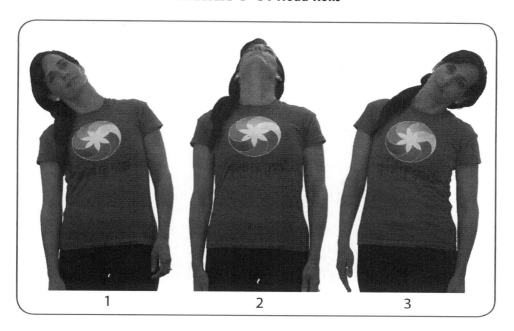

This one is really easy and relaxing, but very important because so much tension gets stored in the neck and shoulder muscles. All that's involved here is slowly rotating your head and neck in as large a circle as you can. Feel the stretching around the entire circle. Go nice a slow, breathing slowly and naturally as you go. Do a few rotations and then reverse direction and go the other way for a few more rotations.

ASANA 5-4: Drinking Rain

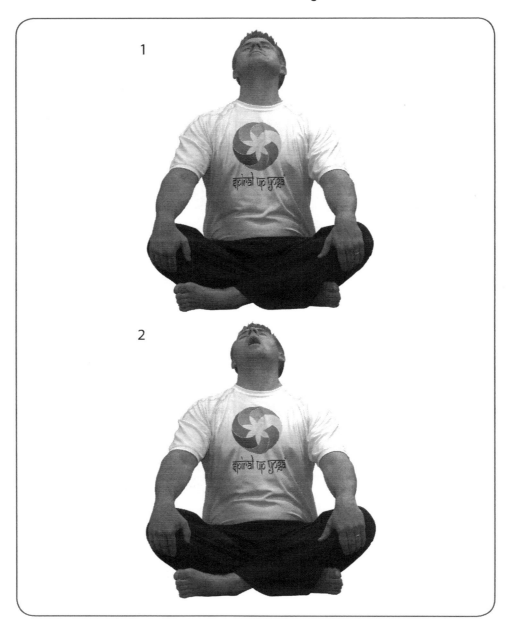

Begin seated cross-legged. Put your hands on your knees and lean your upper body back slightly and drop your head back so your chin is pointing in the air. Open your mouth and drop your lower jaw (Figure 1). Now slowly bring your lower molar teeth up so that they touch your upper jaw molar teeth (Figure 2). You should feel a tightness and stretch in the front of your neck, right in your Fifth Chakra area, as you close your mouth. Keep opening and closing your jaw like this for as long as you like; usually twenty to sixty seconds is fine.

ASANA 5-5: Tuck/Rolling Tuck

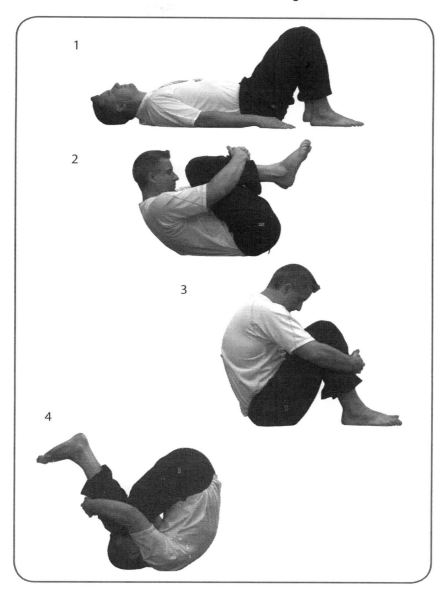

Begin lying on your back with your knees bent and feet flat on floor and arms resting on the ground (Figure 1). Now pull your knees back towards your head and grab around your legs with your arms. Pull your head up towards your chest and tuck your chin in to where it is touching or close to touching your chest (Figure 2). Hold this tuck position for a few counts, breathing naturally through your nose. Now begin the rolling part. Roll forward until your feet are flat on the floor and you are sitting upright (Figure 3). Then roll back along your spine until your head and shoulders are the only thing touching the ground (Figure 4). Continue this back and forth rolling for as long as you like; usually twenty to thirty seconds is fine.

ASANA 5-6: Shoulder Stand/Scissors

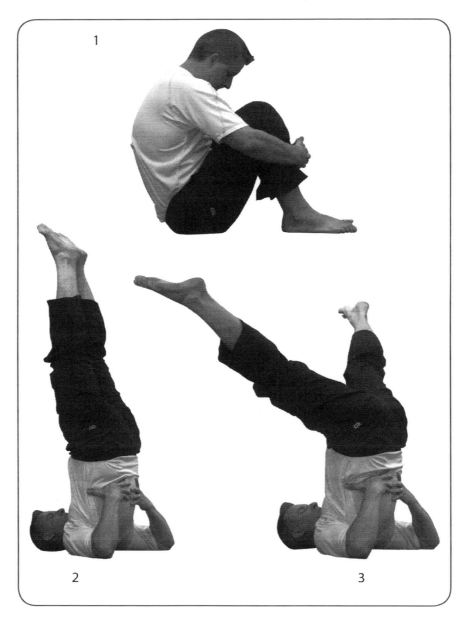

This one is a bit more challenging, but not too much. If you have difficulty sleeping, it's a great one to do before bed. Begin in a seated position, knees bent with your feet flat on the floor (Figure 1). Now roll back onto your shoulders and pull your legs straight up above you. Use the palms of your hands to support your upper back and maintain balance (Figure 1). Hold this position for a few counts and breathe naturally through your nose. Now begin opening and closing your legs like giant scissors (Figure 2). Open and close for a few cycles and then roll back down to your starting position.

ASANA 5-7: Seated Woodchopper

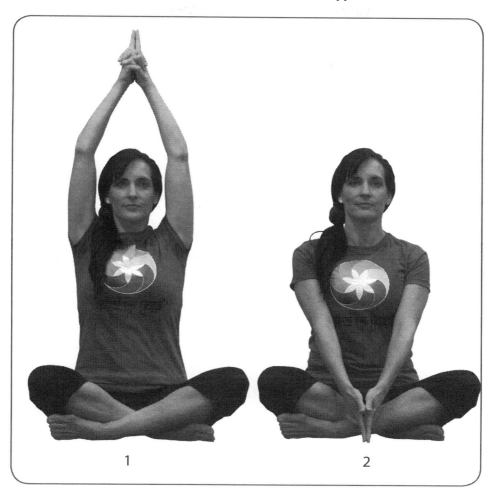

1   2

Begin seated cross-legged. Interlock the fingers of your hands, palms together and raise up your thumbs and index fingers, almost like making a finger gun. Now raise your arms straight up above your head with your index fingers pointing straight up (Figure 1). Imagine you are holding an axe and chopping a block of wood in front of you. Swing your arms down in a downward chopping motion (Figure 2). Continue this up and down chopping motion for as long as you like; usually twenty to sixty seconds is fine. Breathe in as you go up and forcefully exhale through your nose as you chop down.

ASANA 6-1: Bridge

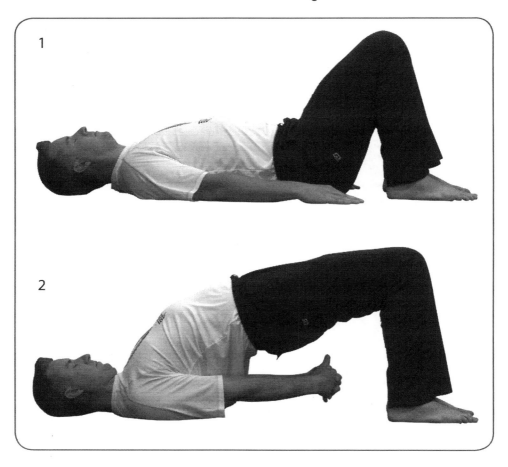

Begin by lying on your back with your knees up and feet flat on the floor (Figure 1). Now press your feet into the ground and raise your hips up so that your weight is supported by your feet and shoulders/upper back. Bring your palms together under your raised back and interlock your fingers (Figure 2). Breath naturally as you hold this pose for as long as you like; usually twenty to sixty seconds is fine.

ASANA 6-2: Cat/Cow

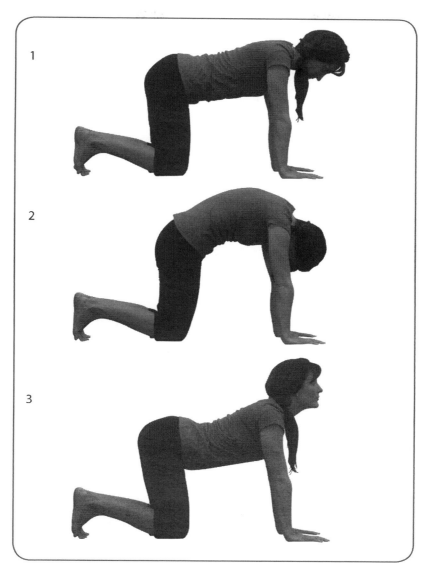

Begin on hands and knees with palms flat on ground, arms below shoulders and knees below hips. Toes should be curled under so they are touching the ground (Figure 1). Now begin alternating slowly between Cat pose and Cow pose. Cat pose is with your back arched up and head tucked down toward your chest (Figure 2). Cow pose is with your back arched down and head up looking straight ahead (Figure 3). Make the motion fluid between the two positions and slowly begin increasing the pace with which you move back and forth between them until you reach a fairly quick pace. Breathe in as you move your head up into Cow pose and out as you move your head down into Cat pose. If you begin to feel lightheaded at all, slow down the pace. Continue moving back and forth between Cat and Cow as long as you like; usually thirty to sixty seconds is fine.

ASANA 6-3: Ratchet Up

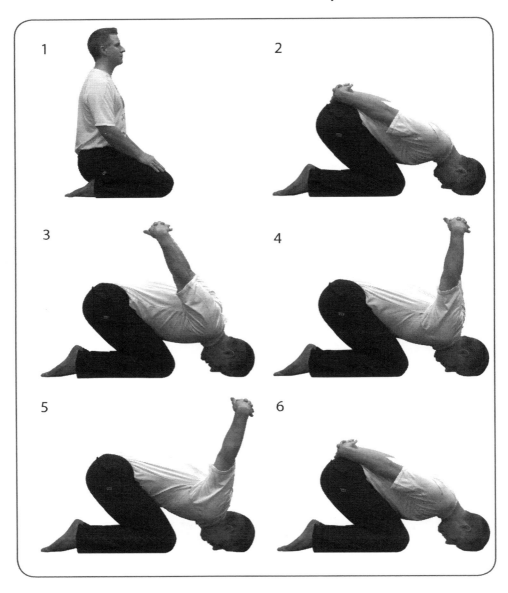

Begin on your knees, sitting back on your feet (Figure 1). Bend forward and place your forehead on the ground while you bring your arms behind your back, palms facing each other and interlock your fingers (Figure 2). Begin a ratcheting up motion with your arms in three increments, taking an in breath with each motion (Figures 2,3,4). Then in one out breath, move your arms back down to where they began where your hands are touching your lower back (Figure 5). Repeat this pattern, three in breaths up, one out breath down and continue for as long as you like; usually thirty to sixty seconds is fine.

ASANA 6-4: Alternating Kneeling Yoga Mudra

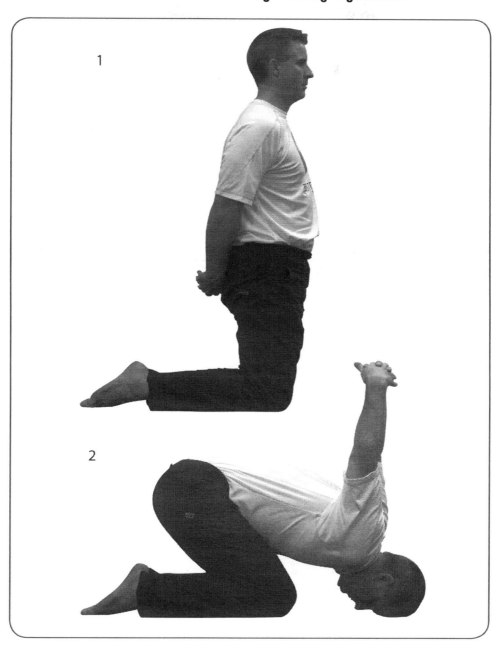

Begin kneeling upright, arms behind back, with fingers interlocked (Figure 1). Bend forward, placing your forehead on the ground and pulling your arms up behind you until they are straight above your head (Figure 2). Begin moving back and forth between these two positions, breathing in as you come up into kneeling position and out as you go down into Yoga Mudra position. Continue as long as you like; usually twenty to sixty seconds is fine.

ASANA 6-5: Baby Pose

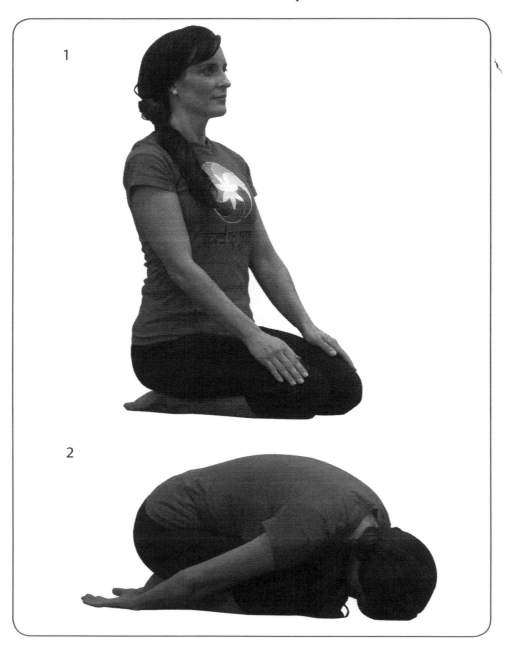

This is an easy, relaxing one. Begin in a kneeling position, sitting back on your feet (Figure 1). Slowly bend forward, placing your forehead on the ground and resting your arms on the floor by your side, palms facing up (Figure 2). In this position, breathe long, deep breaths through your nose and relax as completely as you can. Imagine you are like a baby sleeping in this position without a care in the world, being completely supported. Stay in this position for as long as you like; usually forty to sixty seconds is fine.

ASANA 6-6: Venus Lock

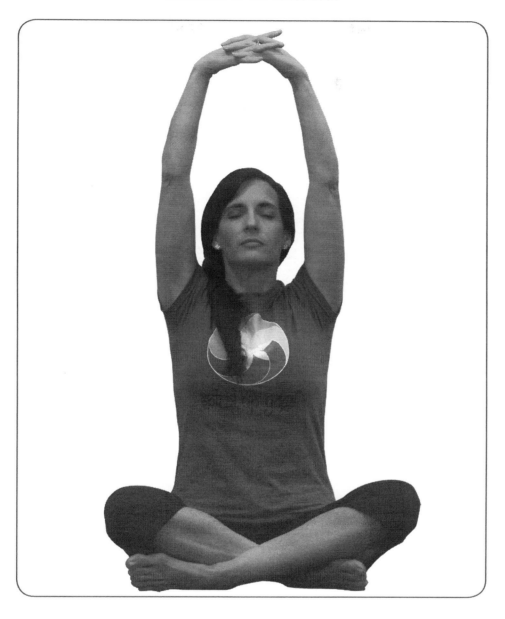

Sit cross-legged and raise your arms above your head, interlocking the fingers with your palms facing down (Figure 1). Close your eyes and turn them up as if looking out your Third Eye (Sixth Chakra), which is at the center of your forehead. Breathe long deep breaths into your lower abdomen and hold in this position for as long as you like; usually thirty to sixty seconds is fine. With your eyes closed, you are focusing your vision inward towards your Third Eye, which sees within and sees through illusions about yourself and your potential that can fool your physical eyes. Imagine seeing through the illusions that are holding you from your potential in some way.

ASANA 6-7: Standing Window of Wisdom

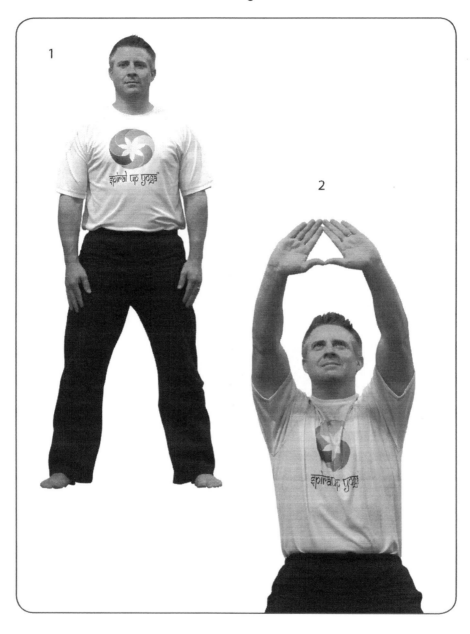

Begin standing with feet hip width apart or just a bit wider (Figure 1). Squat down slightly and raise your arms above and in front of your head, touching your thumbs and index fingers together to make a triangle shape (Figure 2). Focus your gaze in the triangle shaped window you have created with your fingers. Long, deep breathing as you hold this position for as long as you like; usually twenty to thirty seconds is fine. If you want to increase the challenge, squat down further. Imagine that through your window is coming greater wisdom and clarity, flowing into your Third Eye (Sixth Chakra).

ASANA 7-1: Frog

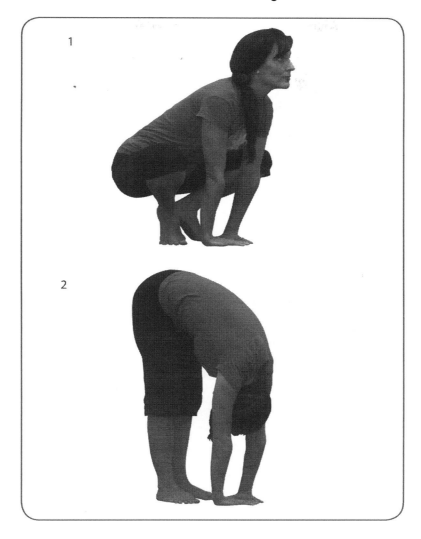

Begin by standing with your heels touching and your feet pointing out about forty-five degrees in each direction so your feet make about a ninety-degree angle. Squat down so your weight is on your toes as your heels come off the ground. Support yourself by putting your hands on the floor and look straight ahead (Figure 1). From this position straighten your legs and put your heels on the ground. Keep your hands on the ground and bend your torso forward, dropping your head and looking toward your shins (Figure 2). Begin moving back and forth between these two positions, breathing in as you straighten your legs and fold forward and out as your bend your legs and unfold. At first you may not be able to keep your hands on the floor as your straighten your legs. That's okay; let your hands rise up as much as they need to so you can straighten your legs. With time and as your flexibility increases, you will be able to keep your hands on the floor as you straighten your legs. Continue alternating between these two positions for twenty to sixty seconds.

ASANA 7-2: Alternating Forward Bend/Fold

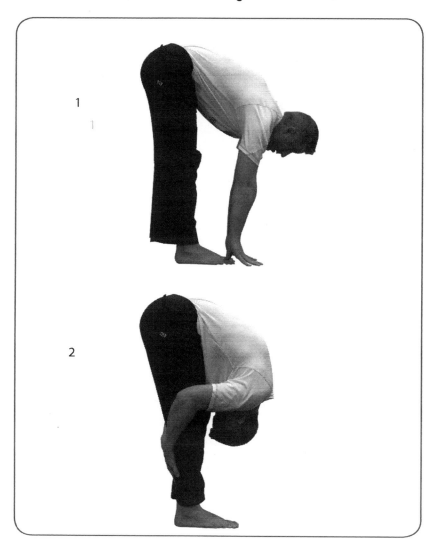

Begin in a standing position. Slowly bend forward while keeping your legs and knees straight, touching as far down your legs or feet or floor as you can. You head should be facing down, eyes looking toward the floor (Figure 1). Now, as you exhale, wrap your arms behind your knees, grabbing your calf muscles with your hands for some leverage. Tuck your head down so you are looking at your legs and fold your torso and legs as close as you can to each other (Figure 2). Slowly begin moving back and forth between these two positions, breathing in as you look towards the ground and out as you look toward your legs, and pull into a deeper fold. Continue for as long as you like; usually twenty to forty seconds is fine. Don't worry if you can't touch the floor or fold back very far, or if you need to bend your knees slightly. Just find the edge of your current flexibility and stay there for now or very gently extend slightly past it.

ASANA 7-3: Downward Dog on Finger and Toe Tips

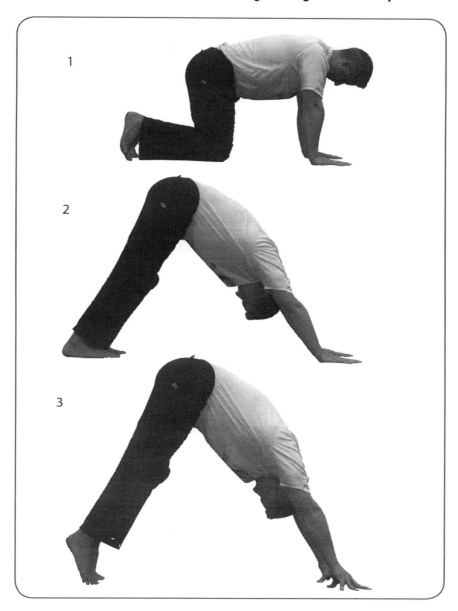

Begin in a kneeling position and move to all fours with arms below shoulders and knees below hips. Curl your toes under and look forward (Figure 1). From here, come up into Downward Dog with feet flat, legs straight, palms flat on floor, arms straight, head down looking toward your knees (Figure 2). Now push up further so that your weight is supported only by your toe tips and finger tips (Figure 3). Hold this position as long as you like; usually ten to twenty seconds is enough. This one is very energizing, literally sending blood flow and energy flow from your core all the way through your finger and toe tips.

ASANA 7-4: Alternating Camel/Bow

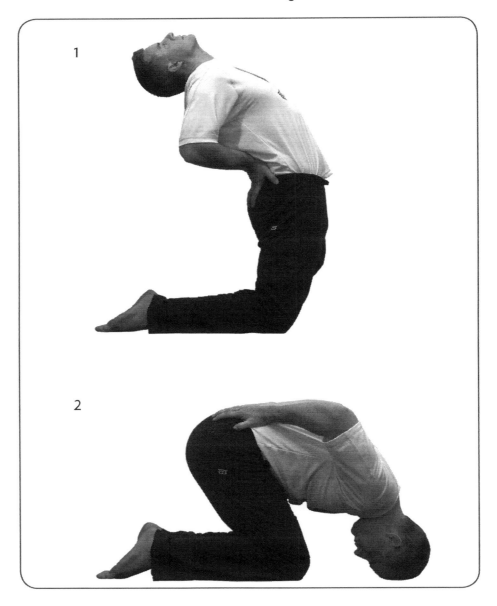

Begin in a kneeling up position, with the tops of your feet flat on the floor. Place the palms of your hands over your kidney area on your lower back and lean backwards until your head is back and your chin is pointing straight up (Figure 1). This is a version of Camel pose. From here move into a Bow pose. Keep your hands where they are and bend your torso forward until the crown of your head is resting on the floor (Figure 2). Begin alternating back and forth between these two poses, breathing in as you move up into Camel and out as you move down into Bow. Continue this motion for as long as you like; usually twenty to sixty seconds is fine.

ASANA 7-5: Head Stand Starter

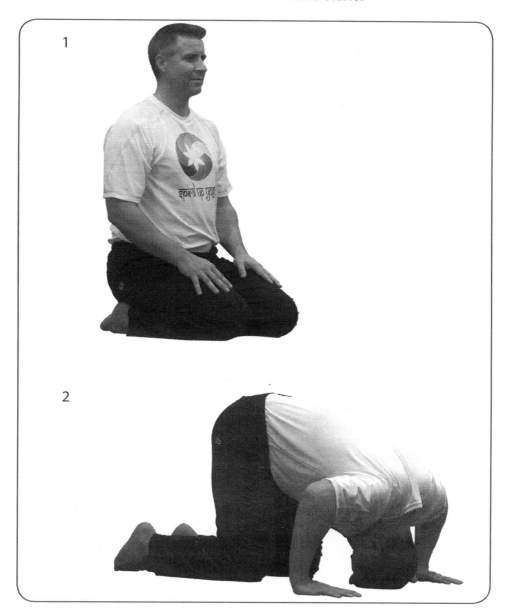

Begin in a kneeling position, sitting back on your feet (Position 1). Come up off your feet and bend forward, placing the crown of your head on the floor and placing the palms of your hands on the floor on either side of your head, about shoulder width apart (Position 2). Hold in this position, as if getting ready to do a headstand. Don't worry, you're not going to do a headstand. This is it; just stay in this position, breathing long deep breaths through your nose. You may want to begin massaging the top of your head some by moving it around the floor a bit. Try moving it forward and back a few inches, then left and right a few inches. Stay in this position as long as you like; usually twenty to sixty seconds is fine.

ASANA 7-6: Seated Spinal Twist

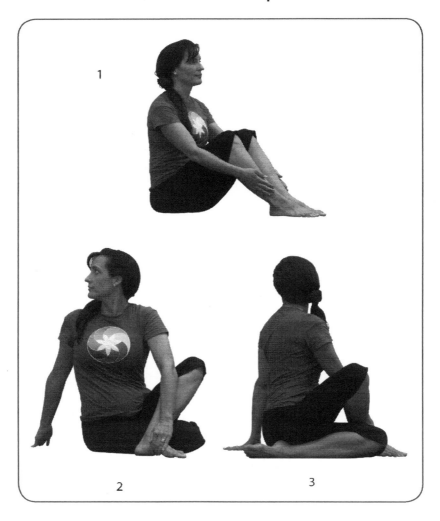

Begin in a seated position with your feet flat on the floor, knees bent, arms gently holding onto your shins (Figure 1). Drop your right leg to the side and move your right foot under your left raised leg until your right knee is pointing straight ahead. Now take your left foot and move it over your right knee so that your left ankle is touching your right leg just above the knee. Place your right arm behind you with your fingers (or palms if you can) on the ground. Place your left arm to the right of your left leg so that your left elbow is touching and pressing against your left knee and your fingertips are touching the floor. Twist your entire torso to the right as you look back over your right shoulder (Figure 2). That was a lot harder to describe in words than it is to actually do; just refer to the picture. At this point your spine should be in a full helix twist, from your tailbone through to the base of your head. Hold this position for several counts as you breathe several long deep breaths. Now release the twist and return to the starting position (Position 1) and then reverse, doing the spinal twist in the opposite (counter-clockwise) direction (Position 3).

ASANA 7-7: Pyramid Crown

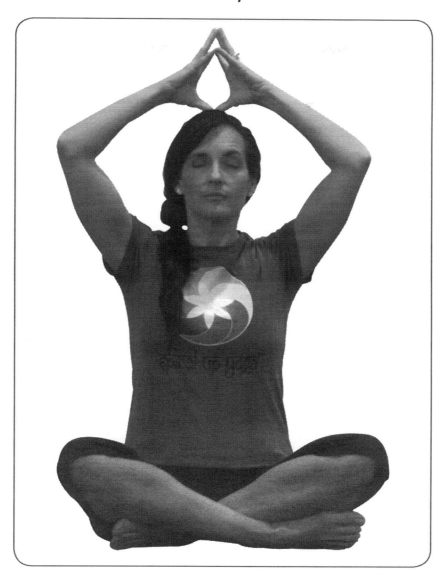

Begin seated cross-legged. With your two hands create a pyramid shape by joining all your fingertips together. Place your thumbs on the crown of your head (Position 1). Stay in this position, breathing long deep breaths for thirty to sixty seconds, or longer if you like. Imagine breathing in pure white energy through the pyramid/prism of your hands into the crown of your head (Seventh Chakra) as you breathe in, and as you breathe out imagine that white light is split into the seven colors of the rainbow, which are not coincidentally the same colors of the seven chakras. Red at your First Chakra, orange at your Second Chakra, yellow at your Third Chakra, green at your Fourth Chakra, blue at your Fifth Chakra, indigo at your Sixth Chakra, and purple at your Seventh Chakra.

34

FREQUENTLY ASKED QUESTIONS

Q: How do I know this system will work for me?

A: You can't know until you test it. It won't take too long before you'll know. I recommend you give it at least three or four weeks of testing and then see how you feel compared to before. Many will realize it in much less time. If you don't think it works for you, don't do it. All you're out is the tiny cost of buying the book.

Q: Do I need any special clothing, mats, or equipment to practice Spiral Up Yoga?

A: No. All you need is you and a few square feet of space. You don't need to wear any special clothing or shoes. I do most of my practice barefoot and in my pj's in my own bedroom. A few of the tools, such as aromatherapy oils and tuning forks, do require a one-time purchase. These are optional, and you can add them when you want. I personally love these other tools and build them into my daily practice, but you can choose if and when that is right for you.

Q: If I miss a day (or more), do I start from the First Chakra day again?

A: No. Just pick up on the day that you're on. If today is Wednesday and you haven't done anything since last Friday, just do the Wednesday (Third Chakra) practices. Keeping the days of the week tied to the chakras is the only real structure to the Spiral Up Yoga system. Stick with it so that it soon becomes a healthy habit. After a while, if it's Wednesday, you know exactly what types of things to do to strengthen the Third Chakra. It's better to be inconsistent, but to still do it when you remember, than to get frustrated and quit altogether.

Q: Is the Spiral Up Yoga system all I will ever need in terms of self-care of body, mind, and soul?

A: Spiral Up Yoga is a wonderful foundational practice of self-care for body, mind, and soul that takes only about five minutes a day to practice. It is not designed as a complete replacement for other forms of exercise, nutrition, or spiritual nurturing. You can keep doing anything you're already doing. There is nothing about Spiral Up Yoga that would interfere with anything else you're already doing or might want to add later. Just let this become your five-minutes-a-day foundation to which you can add anything else as you choose. I still do longer yoga sets at times, as well as go on walks, runs, bike rides, swims, etc. I also still practice meditation, prayer, and the reading of sacred texts and inspirational books. But even if I don't fit any other form of self-care in, when I do my Spiral Up Yoga practice, I do something, no matter how small, to strengthen that day's chakra – even if it only takes one minute.

Q: If I have some chronic physical body conditions, is it because I have neglected my energy body and chakras, and if so, is strengthening them all I need to do to heal myself?

A: If you have a chronic physical body condition that has developed over time, it does mean that you have neglected the care of your energy body and chakras, as no chronic physical body symptom can exist without a corresponding weakness or blockage in the more subtle energy body. Your treatment of your symptom should include, but not be limited to, doing things to strengthen your energy body and chakras. Add that to any treatment recommended by your medical practitioner. That way you will not only improve the particular physical body condition that is currently showing up, but you will be restoring your chakras so that the next physical body symptom is less likely to show up.

Q: After a while, won't I have gotten all the good I'm going to get out of this practice?

A: No. There is no limit to the good you can get out of your own Spiral Up Yoga practice. The tools have unlimited possibility. Not only can you put together different tools, but you can go deeper into each one or become more mindful and aware as you perform each one. In addition, you can add anything you come across that helps you strengthen your chakras.

Q: Can I injure myself doing Spiral Up Yoga?

A: You can potentially injure yourself doing any form of exercise, even just taking a walk. I ruptured a disc in my back one morning just getting out of bed (before I started practicing yoga). The asanas are the only physical exercise in the Spiral Up Yoga system. Use your judgment. Do not push past your physical body's current limits, or you could injure yourself. Respect where your body is right now and know that with time and consistency, it will improve. You may only be able to touch your knees now, but before too long, you could be touching your toes, and then the floor.

Q: What style of yoga do you teach as part of Spiral Up Yoga?

A: The asanas that I teach come from various styles or forms of yoga. It isn't from any one official style, but a collection of asanas that I have personally experimented with and found to have a particularly focused effect on a specific chakra. The asanas I include in this book and on the website are only a few of the many different asanas available. I encourage you to try these, but if you are already a practitioner of other styles of yoga that you like, bring additional asanas of your choosing into your practice. This is your practice, not mine. It is meant to be custom created by you, for you.

Q: What qualifies you to be a teacher of yoga. What certifications do you have?

A: The only thing that qualifies me is my decision to share with others what I've discovered for myself. This is a perfect example of something called "self-authorization," which I highly recommend because it's something that so often gets beaten out of us as children and teenagers. We start believing the illusion that we need someone else's permission to do what we want to do. We need a publisher to say "yes" to our book, and we need a boss to say "yes" to hire us. We need a distributor to say "yes" to carrying our product. Of course there are a few professions where certification is needed, like to become a medical doctor or lawyer or airline pilot, but for 95% of what you want to do, the only person's permission you need is yours. What do you authorize yourself to do?

Q: Where can I learn more about your training, coaching, and speaking?

A: All the additional resources, training, coaching, and speaking that I offer can be found at www.spiralupyoga.com.

Q: How can I connect with other people who are practicing Spiral Up Yoga? Do you have a Spiral Up Yoga community online?

A: Yes. Join our Spiral Up Community online at www.spiralupyoga.com, where you can support and learn from each other. It's free to join.

14503043R00126

Made in the USA
Lexington, KY
02 April 2012